Pregnancy Cookbook

What to Eat and How to Cook During Your Pregnancy - The Go-To Cookbook for Pregnant Ladies

BY: Ivy Hope

Copyright © 2020 by Ivy Hope

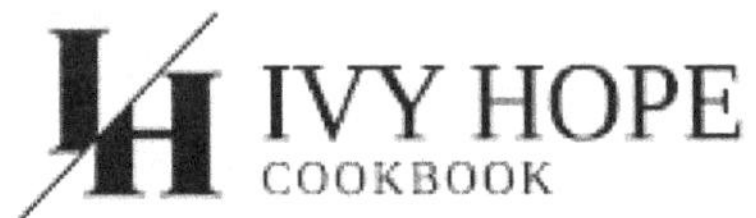

Copyright/License Page

Table of Contents

Introduction

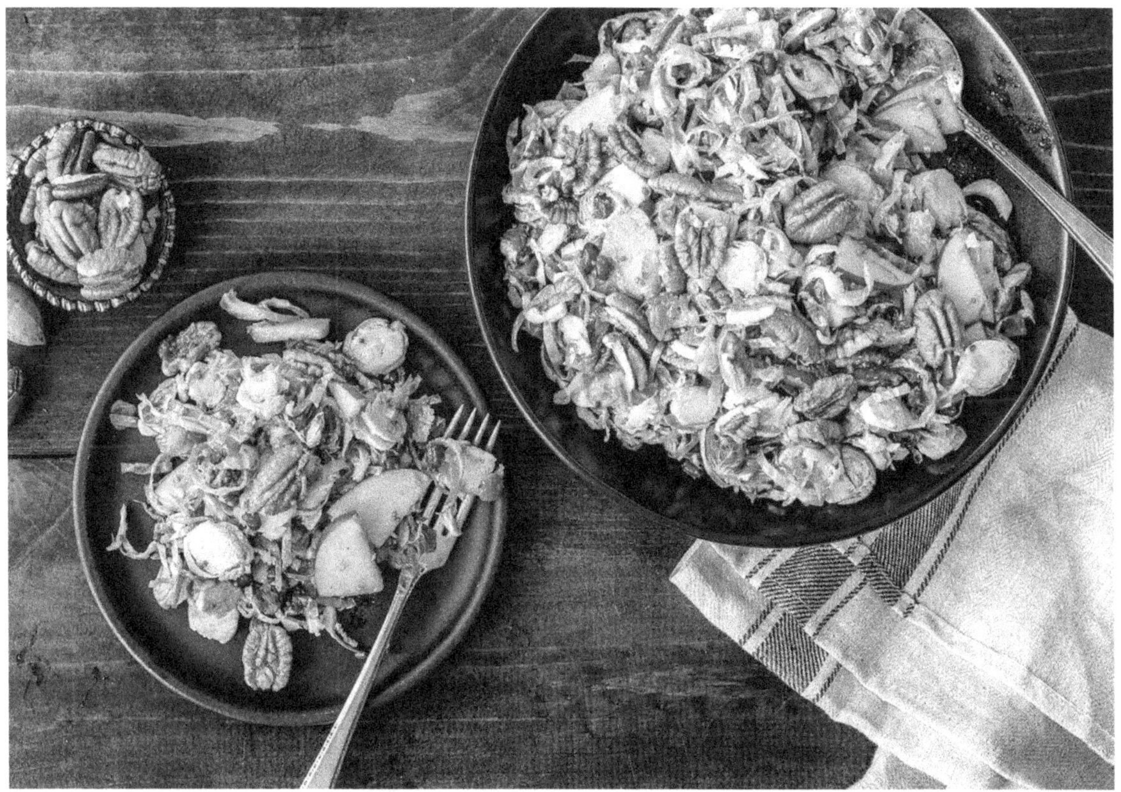

We will only suggest some foods we know that are safe when we present our recipes. In this chapter, however, we feel like it is crucial to tell you what foods you should avoid as a pregnant woman.

- Any raw or uncooked food, such as raw eggs and sushi. Be particularly careful when cooking your meats, burger meat, and chicken to make sure it is cooked thoroughly.
- Not only should you avoid sushi, but any raw fish. Always avoid fish that contain high levels of mercury.

- Raw eggs are notably found in homemade salad dressing, sauces, mayonnaise, custards. So, always read ingredients on labels carefully and avoid these foods when you go out as well.

- Avoid caffeine, soda, coffee, and tea. If you can't live without coffee, please limit your consumption to a cup a day, and wait until your first trimester is over.

- It's not time to party! Avoid drinking alcohol. It is not safe to drink alcohol during your pregnancy, period. You should also exempt yourself from drinking if you are breastfeeding after delivery.

- Avoid any organ meats, such as liver, stomachs, brain, and more.

- In addition, avoid any meat spreads or pates since they are usually made with meat organs or can contain a certain percentage.

- Make sure you wash your product carefully before using them raw or cooked.

- Deli meats should also be avoided; they can contain bacteria listeria, which can be very dangerous for you.

- As much as you need your calcium, you should avoid certain types of cheese during pregnancy and the soft cheese that is. For example, brie, camembert, Feta, or Queso should be avoided.

Now our goal is not to scare you or make you worry extra, but it is also known that some specific foods could even cause miscarriages, so please be extra careful. Among these foods, we should list the sprouted potatoes, unpasteurized milk, raw eggs, smoked seafood, papaya, some meat livers.

1. Freshly baked nuts bread

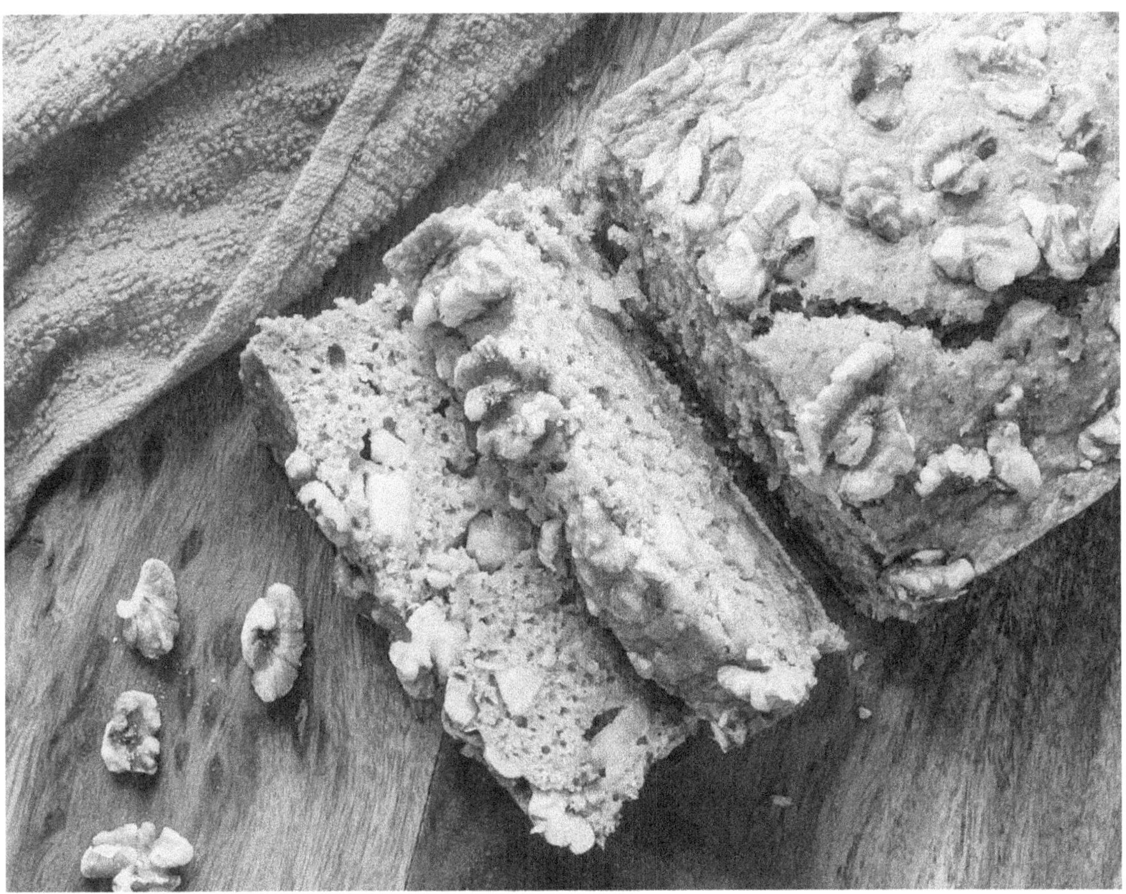

Nuts are not only yummy in a break like this one, but they are very healthy for pregnant women. Apparently, they can contribute to reducing blood pressure when high and reduce diabetes in some cases. Nuts are high in fiber, so healthy bowel movements are appreciated while pregnant. Eat them in recipes or as an afternoon snack!

Ingredients:

- 2 cups all-purpose flour
- 1 cup crushed walnuts
- 1 large egg
- ¼ cup whole milk
- 1 tsp. baking soda
- 1 tsp. baking power
- ½ cup brown sugar
- 1 tsp. cinnamon
- Pinch salt

Servings: 6-10

Preparation time: 1 hour

Method:

Preheat the oven first to 350 degrees F.

Grease a loaf pan and set aside.

In a large mixing bowl, combine the dry ingredients together: flour, sugar, cinnamon, salt, baking powder and baking soda.

Add the milk, nuts and the egg next and combine again with wooden spoon.

Dump the mixture into the pan and bake for 45 minutes.

Wait until the bread cools down and slice.

2. Warm hearty beef stew

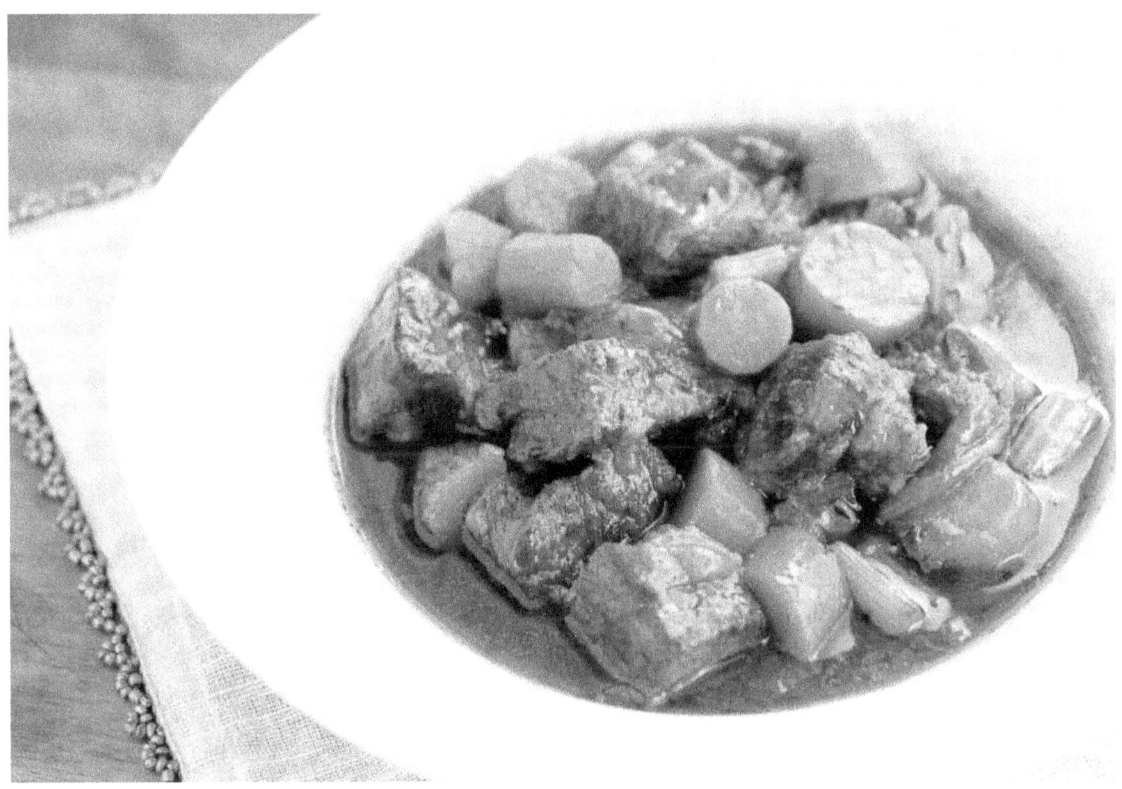

Not only a stew can contain so many vegetables and your intake of proteins for the day, but if you use red meat to prepare, here are the extra benefits you will add to your diet. Red meat is important to your blood supply mommies to be. Therefore, adding red meat will help bring extra oxygen to you and your baby while he is taking more and more space in your belly. You can, however, choose some lean red meat.

Ingredients:

- 2 pounds stew beef (chuck roast)
- 5 cups beef broth
- ¼ cup flour
- Unsalted butter
- 3 chopped celery stalks
- 2 sliced medium peeled carrots
- 1 small chopped yellow onion
- 1 Tbsp., minced garlic
- ½ tsp. dried basil
- ½ tsp. dried oregano
- ½ tsp. ground cumin
- ½ tsp. cayenne pepper
- ½ tsp. salt

Servings: 4-8

Preparation time: 1 hour

Method:

In a large saucepan, heat the butter. Place all pieces of beef in the flour and make sure they are slightly covered.

Cook the beef for 5 minutes in the butter, stirring often.

Remove and set aside.

Add a little butter and all the vegetables. Sautéed the veggies for about 6-7 minutes.

Add the broth, the semi-cooked beef and all seasonings.

Let them beef stew cook for about 45 minutes or more.

You could very well make this recipe in your slow cooker. Instead of using the saucepan, you would still sautéed meat and veggies but dump all ingredients ion the crockpot for 5 hours on low temperature.

3. Strawberries simple smoothie

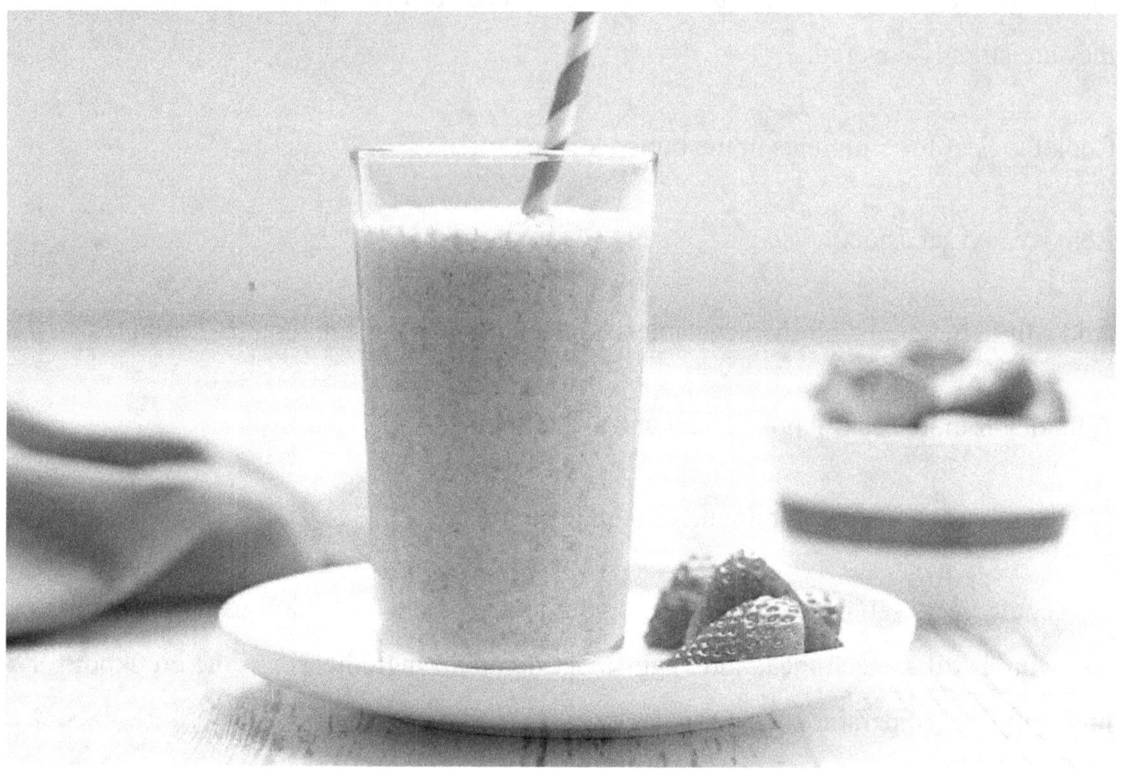

All berries are recommended during pregnancy. Here, we just happened to choose strawberries, but you could prepare this smoothie with any of your favorite berries. The berries are high in antioxidants, fiber, folate, and vitamin C, all essentials for you and baby.

Ingredients:

- 1 cup yoghurt
- ½ cup 2% milk
- 1 cup fresh strawberries
- 1/2 tsp. vanilla extract

Servings: 1

Preparation time: 5 min

Method:

Place all the ingredients in the blender's container and activate until the mixture is completely smooth.

Serve in a tall glass with or without a straw.

4. A special banana soup

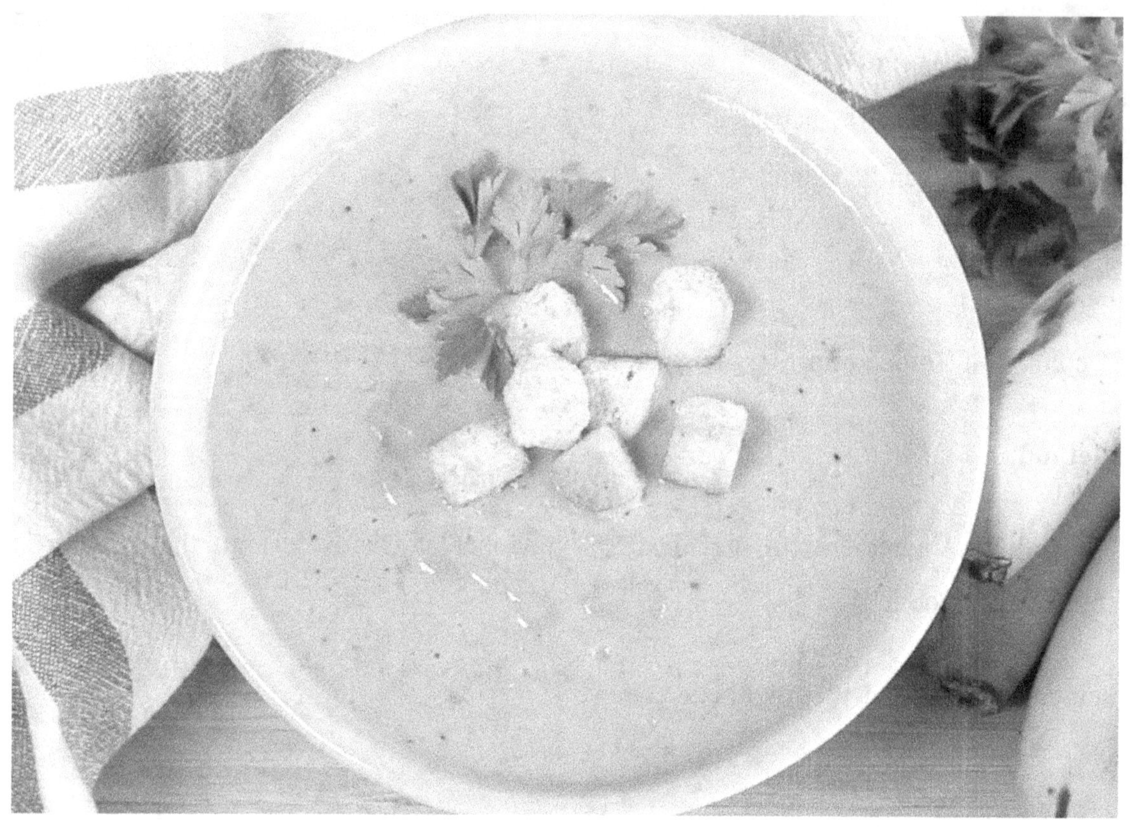

A banana is certainly an easy to-go snack and a healthy one. As a pregnant woman, you can benefit from its excellent source of potassium. In addition, bananas are rich in vitamin B-6, vitamin C, and fiber. This soup is definitely very different, but different can be good, so you don't get bored with routines.

Ingredients

- 1 Tbsp. unsalted butter
- 2 large ripe bananas
- 4 cups low sodium chicken broth
- 1-cup coconut milk
- 1 small chopped sweet onion
- ½ tsp. cinnamon
- ½ tsp. rosemary
- Salt, pepper
- 1 Tbsp. coconut palm sugar

Servings: 3-4

Preparation time: 45 min

Method:

In a small skillet, heat the butter and cook the onion for 5 minutes. Set aside.

Place in the blender's container, the banana, coconut milk, cooked onion and activate until the texture is smooth.

In a medium saucepan, heat the chicken broth and add the sugar and spices. Stir often to make sure the sugar dissolves.

Add the banana mixture and combine.

Keep on low temperature for 40 minutes to make sure all flavors blend well.

Serve warm, enjoy and surprise your guests!

5. Blueberries cobbler for you

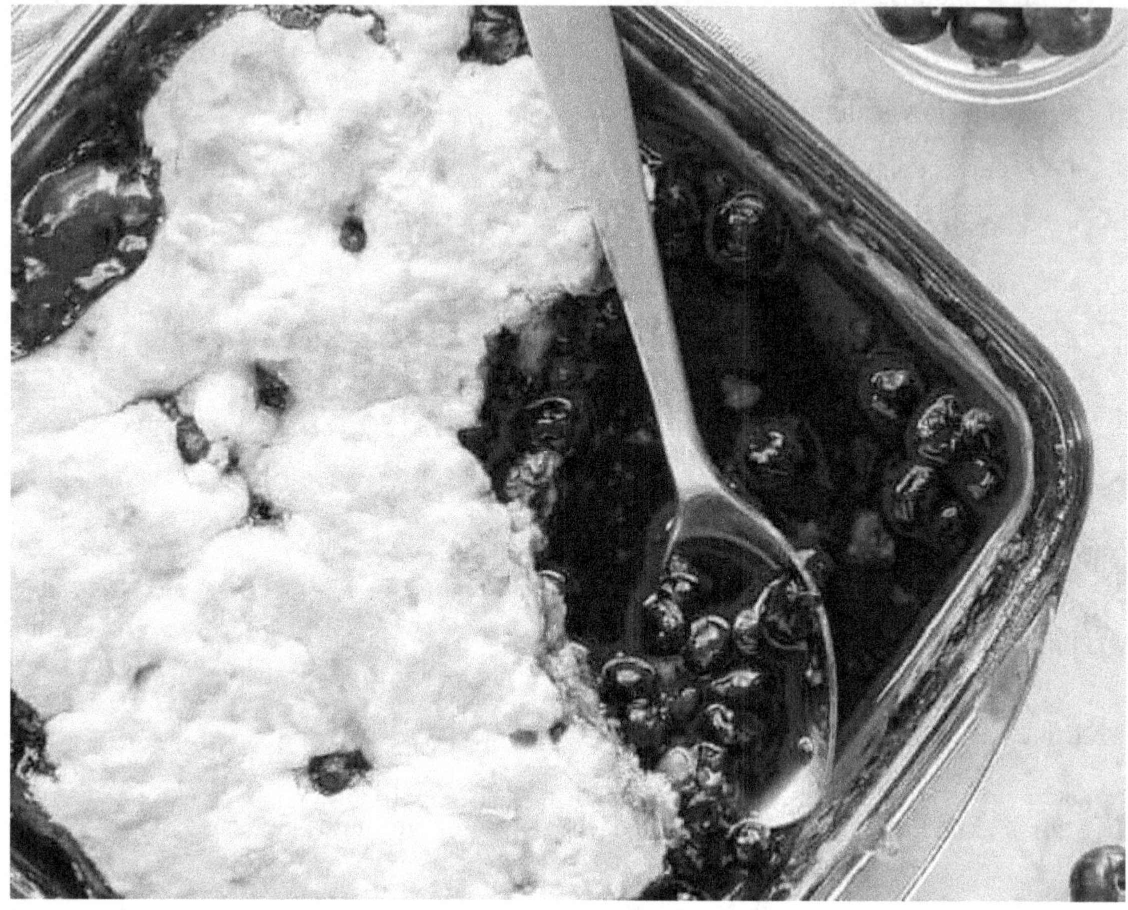

As we stated before, all berries are beneficial to your health, especially when you are pregnant. Blueberries being very high in antioxidants are known to help memory and keep your body rejuvenate. Again, this recipe could very well be well prepared with strawberries, blackberries, or raspberries, your choice. I have used strawberries and rhubarb before to make this recipe, and it was sublime!

Ingredients:

- 3 cups fresh blueberries
- 1 cup rice flour
- 1 cup coconut flour
- 1 tsp. baking soda
- 1 tbsp. baking powder
- 3 Tbsp. maple syrup
- ¼ cup coconut milk
- 2 medium eggs
- Pinch cinnamon
- Pinch nutmeg
- Pinch salt

Servings: 6-8

Preparation time: 55 min

Method:

Preheat the oven to 350 degrees F.

Grease a rectangle baking pan and set aside. You can also use parchment paper if you prefer.

Make sure you wash carefully the fresh blueberries and drain well. Set aside.

In a large mixing bowl, combine the dry ingredients: baking powder, spices, flours, and baking soda.

In a different bowl, combine the wet ones: eggs, milk, maple syrup.

Dump the wet ingredients in the dry mixture. Combine well.

Finally add the blueberries to the mixture and combine gain carefully.

Dump the mixture into the baking dish,

Bake for 45 minutes.

Serve with plain yoghurt.

6. Yogurt based yummy dip

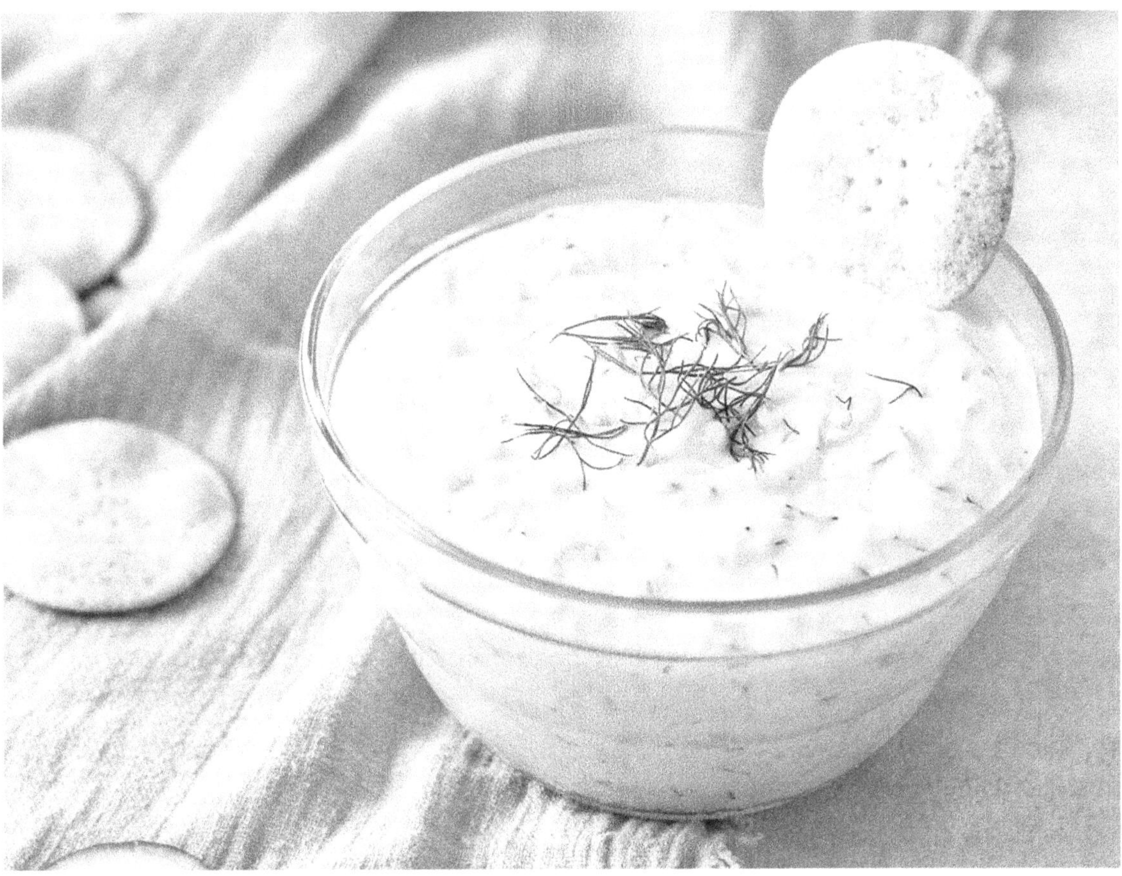

We insist that calcium is important in your pregnancy diet. You will find calcium in yoghurt, mail, and cheese. Yogurt will also provide you some probiotics, helping your need for a significant intake in probiotics and proteins. This dip will keep well for about a week.

Ingredients:

- 2 cups Greek plain yoghurt
- 1 Tbsp. minced fresh chives
- 1 tbsp. minced garlic
- 1 Tbsp. minced fresh parsley
- Pinch cayenne pepper
- Pinch salt

Servings: 8-12

Preparation time: 10 min

Method:

Make sure you wash and drain the fresh herbs carefully before chopping them.

In a medium serving bowl, combining all the ingredients.

Taste the dip and adjust seasonings to your pleasing.

Use with raw veggies or whole-wheat pita bread.

7. Bakes key west style salmon

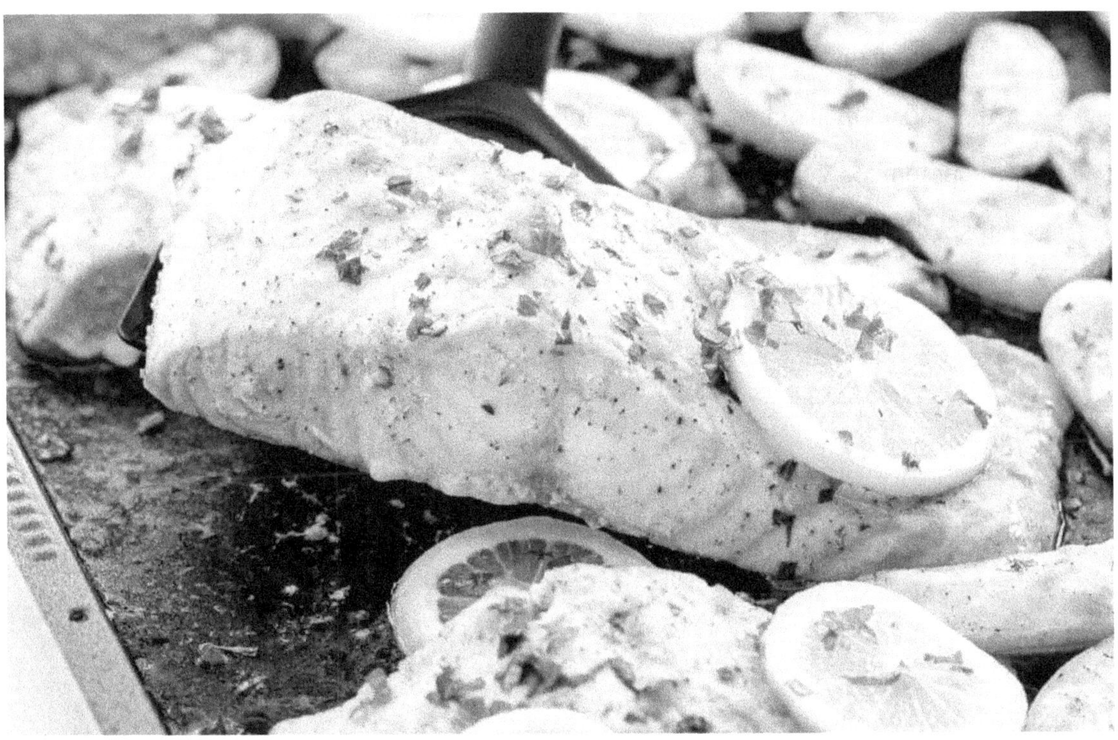

Salmon is one of the healthiest fish you can include in your diet when you are pregnant. Make sure you pick very fresh fish and cook it thoroughly before serving. You will then benefit from omega 3 fatty acid, which is primordial for your child's development. Wait until you taste this particular recipe, it's delicious! You could use the same ingredients and make some sautéed key west shrimp in a wok or skillet next time!

Ingredients:

- 4 salmon fillets
- 2 tbsp. lime juice
- 1 tbs. red pepper flakes
- 1 tbsp. minced garlic
- 2 tbsp. olive oil
- 1 Tbsp. fresh minced cilantro
- ½ tsp. sea salt

Servings: 4

Preparation time: 50 min

Method:

Preheat the oven to 350 degrees F.

Grease a rectangle baking dish and set aside.

In a small mixing bowl, combine the oil, spices and cilantro with lime juice.

Place the 4 fillets skin down on the dish.

Use a cooking brush to spread the oily mixture on each fillet.

Bake in the oven for 25 minutes.

Serve with lime wedges and your favorites veggies.

8. Stir fried greens

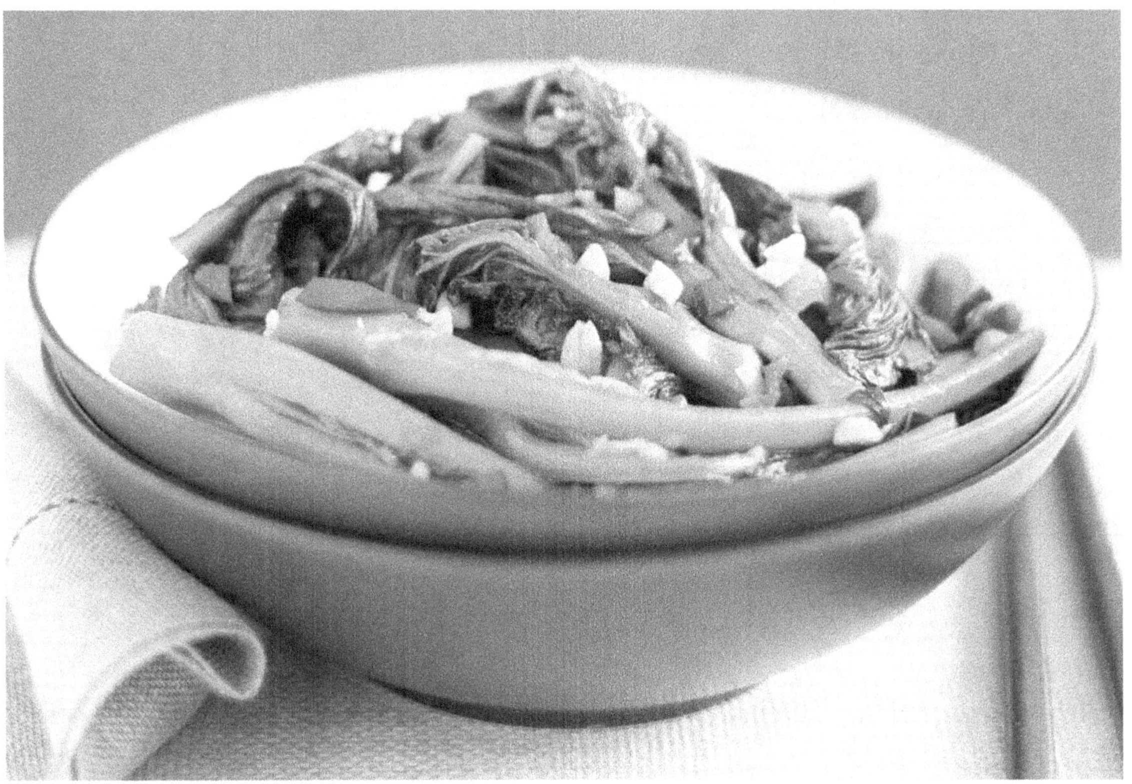

The greener, the better! You should definitely favor dark green vegetables in your diet while you are pregnant. Dark green vegetables, like kale, are rich in vitamins A, C, K, iron, and vitamin B. This will strengthen and your baby brain's development. If you are not a big fan of kale, use spinach or collar greens.

Ingredients:

- 4-6 cups fresh kale
- 1 Tbsp. minced garlic
- ½ tsp. onion powder
- ½ tsp. cayenne pepper
- Salt
- Olive oil
- 1 Tbsp. lemon juice

Servings: 3-4

Preparation time: 10 min

Method:

Kale is an inquired taste. I think adding the spices and lemon juice makes it much tastier.

Wash the kale thoroughly as it often contains dirt and drain well.

Heat the oil in large skillet and cook the garlic for a few minutes before adding the kale.

Add also all seasonings and lemon juice.

Stir for the next 5 minutes.

Serve right away when warm as a side dish or a mid-afternoon green snack.

9. Beans skillet casserole

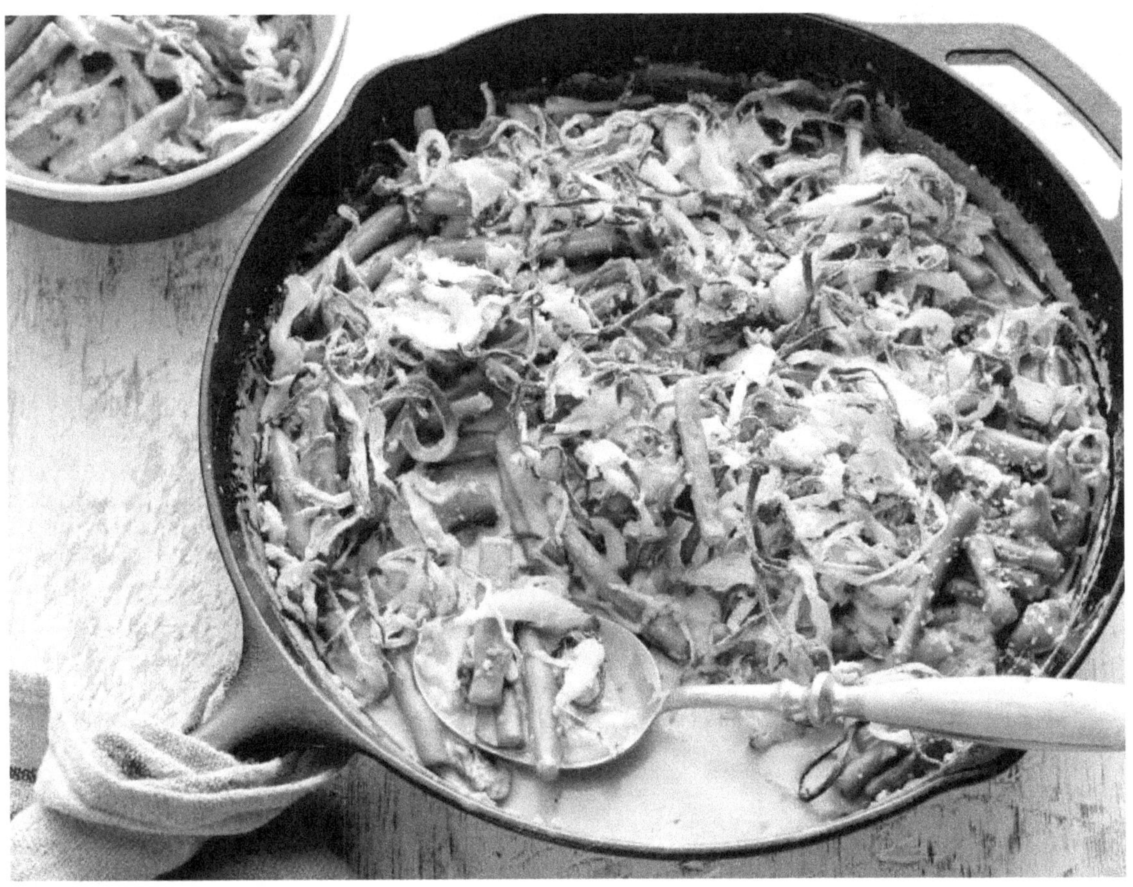

Should you eat beans while you are pregnant? The answer is yes! They are filled with proteins and folic acid, potassium, and more. It also provides you a nice source of fiber, and as you may be constipated during pregnancy, it can help with keeping you regular.

Ingredients:

- 1 medium chopped yellow onion
- 1 tbsp. minced garlic
- 1 minced red bell pepper
- 1 minced green bell pepper
- 2 cans red kidney beans
- 1 can white kidney beans
- 2 cups vegetables broth
- ¼ cup sour cream
- ½ tsp. cumin
- Salt, black pepper
- Olive oil

Servings: 4-6

Preparation time: 45 min

Method:

Use a large skillet or saucepan for this recipe.

Heat the oil on medium temperature and cook the garlic, onion and bell peppers for 10 minutes or so.

Meanwhile, rinsed and drained all the beans very well.

Add to the cooked veggies along with the broth and spices.

Stir and dump the sour cream next.

Stir again until all ingredients all well combined.

Let the recipe simmer for at least 30-45 minutes before serving.

Serves well with corn bread.

10. Easy stuffed avocados

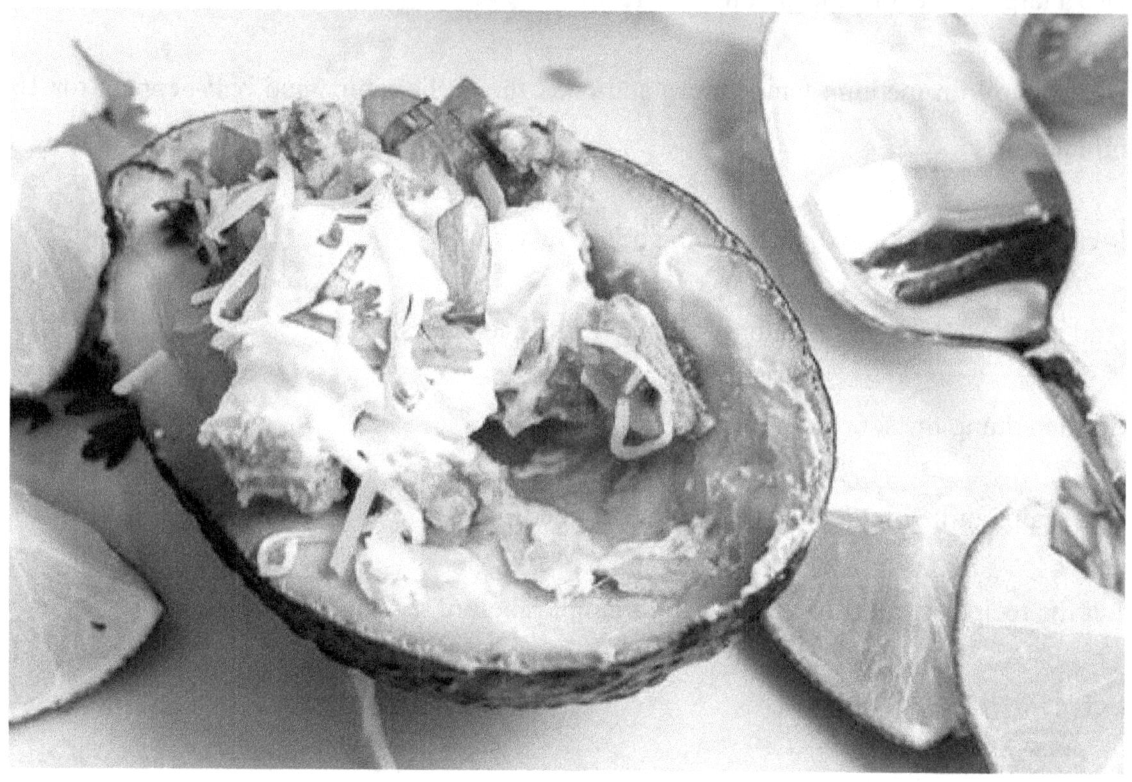

Avocados being a fruit, it is recommended to eat more fruits during pregnancy than normally. Avocados are rich in good fats and folate, which you cannot ever get enough. Be creative and add them to your salads, sandwiches, and more.

Ingredients:

- 4 medium avocados
- 1 pound ground turkey meat
- 1 cup fresh diced tomatoes
- 1 sliced zucchini
- 1 Tbsp. minced garlic
- 1 Tbsp. avocado oil
- ½ cup shredded Cheddar cheese
- 1 tsp. chili powder

Servings: 8-12

Preparation time: 50 min

Method:

Preheat the oven to 400 degrees F.

Grease a square baking dish and set aside.

In a skillet, you will want to cook the veggies first.

Heat some oil and cook the garlic and zucchini for 5 minutes. Set aside.

In the same skillet, cook the turkey meat, adding seasonings.

Remove all excess fat and add in a mixing bowl.

Cut each avocado in halves lengthwise. Remove the seed and remove some of the avocado flesh on each side.

Place the avocados halves on the baking dish.

Add the cooked veggies to the meat, as well as all the avocado flesh. Combine well.

Stuff each avocado with the mixture and top if off with cheese.

Place in the oven for 20 minutes or until the cheese has melted.

11. Delightful spinach omelet

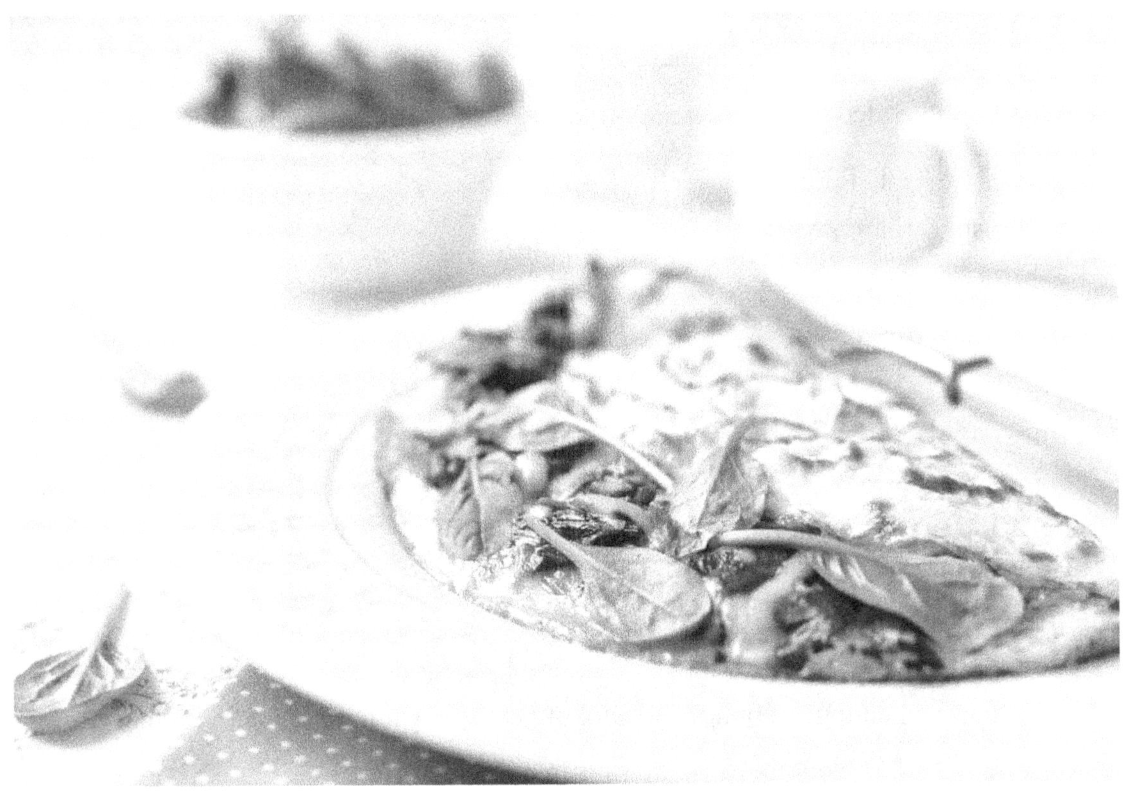

Eggs and spinach are a terrific combination; they are both recommended during pregnancy. As mentioned before, spinach, this dark leafy vegetable if full of iron and folate and it can directly affect your child's development. By eating spinach, you can ensure your child gets a healthy brain and spine.

Ingredients:

- 4 large eggs
- 3 cups fresh baby spinach leaves
- 1 cup shredded Swiss cheese
- Salt, black pepper
- ½ tsp. garlic powder
- 1 tbsp. butter
- 2 Tbsp. Whole milk

Servings: 4

Preparation time: 15 min

Method:

I usually start by heating the butter and cooking the spinach for a few minutes only.

Meanwhile, or even before, I whisk together the eggs, cheese, milk and seasonings.

Add the egg's mixture with the spinach and continue cooking.

Stir to make sure all ingredients mix week and cook until eggs are done.

Serve right away with maybe a side of mild salsa or hot sauce, if you are a fan.

12. Dried apricots fun bites

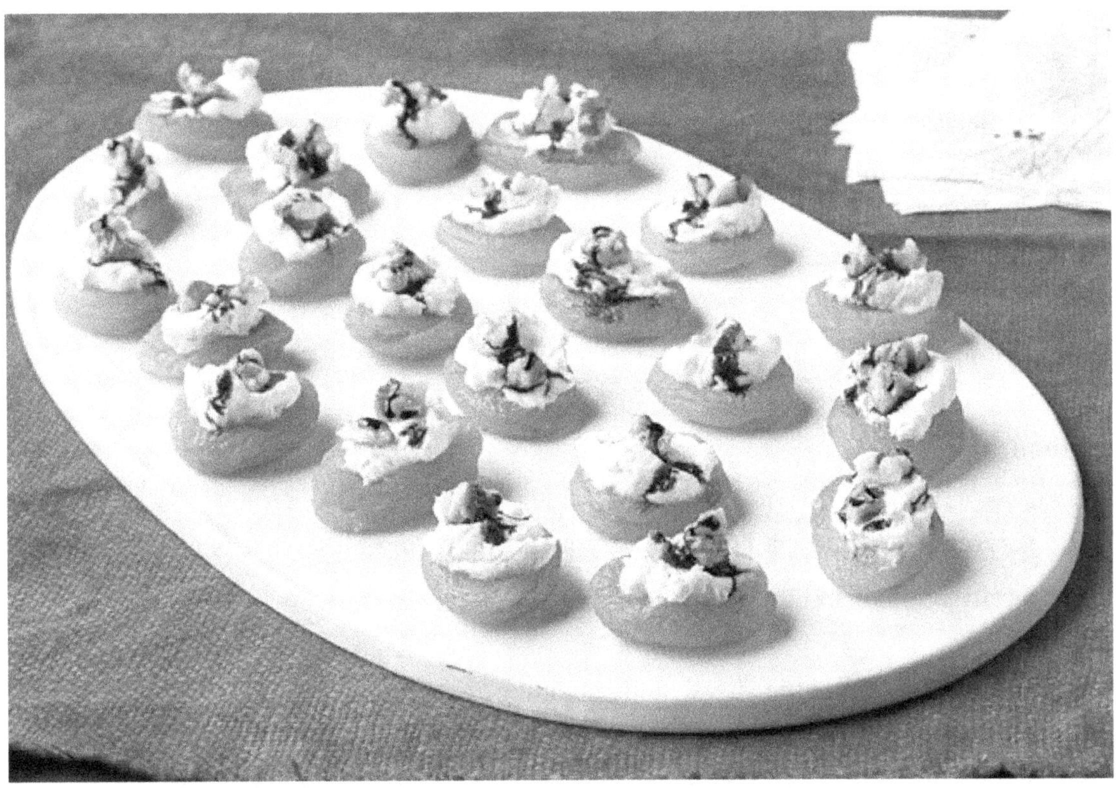

These bites are definitely cute, and fun to make and eat. In addition, as a pregnant woman, here is why apricots and most dried fruits are super good for you. They contain potassium, calcium, and magnesium, along with almost 10% of your daily iron recommended intake. So, keep them in your purse, your gym bag, or at the office, they are such healthy snacks!

Ingredients:

- 1 bag large dried apricots (24 +)
- 1 package plain cream cheese, room temperature
- 1 cup pecans
- 1 tsp. cinnamon

Servings: 6-12

Preparation time: 20 min

Method:

Get a serving plate out or a container if you are preparing these snacks ahead, you will want to refrigerate them until ready to serve.

In a small bowl combine the cheese and cinnamon.

Take one apricot at a time, spread a generous portion of the cheese and then top it off with a pecan.

Repeat the operation until all the apricots are garnished or until you run out of ingredients.

These bites are also very children friendly, so if you are already a mommy, make these at your next child's party, it will be a success for sure!

13. Almond butter, berries in a mug

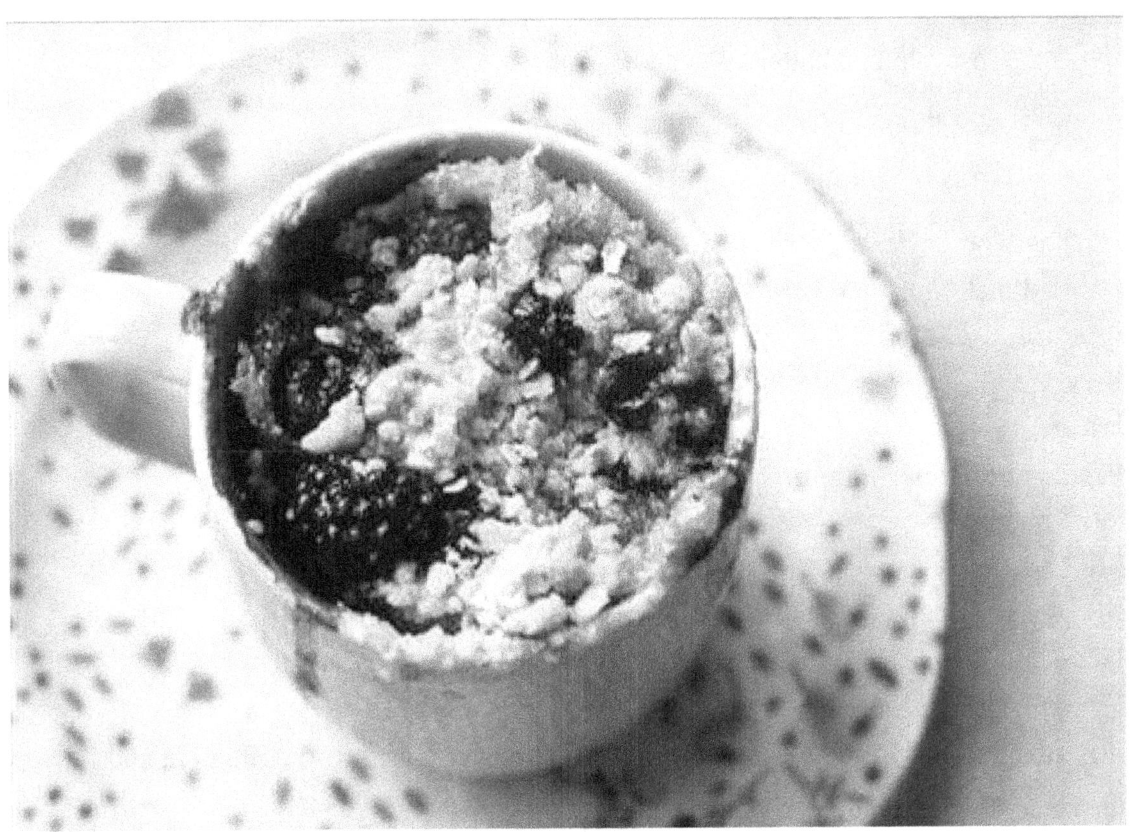

Either you decide to eat your nuts as is or use them in a butter form; you will find many benefits during pregnancy. Seeds and nuts offer you a wonderful source of healthy fats, and they add such yummy taste to make of your original recipes. Remember this recipe because your children-to-be will certainly love it as well!

Ingredients:

- 3 Tbsp. blackberries
- 1 Tbsp. almond butter
- ½ cup almond flour
- 1 Tbsp. brown sugar
- ¼ tsp. baking powder
- Pinch cinnamon

Servings: 1

Preparation time: 12 min

Method:

I love how simple this single portion or recipe is.

It is also nutritious and delicious, so go ahead and get your favorite mug out and line up the listed ingredients on the counter.

In your mug, combine all the dry ingredients. Stir to mix.

Add the blackberries.

Place the mug in the microwave for 1.5 minute on high temperature.

Remove and let cool down a little and serve with your favorite yoghurt on top.

14. Traditional devils eggs but with no mayonnaise

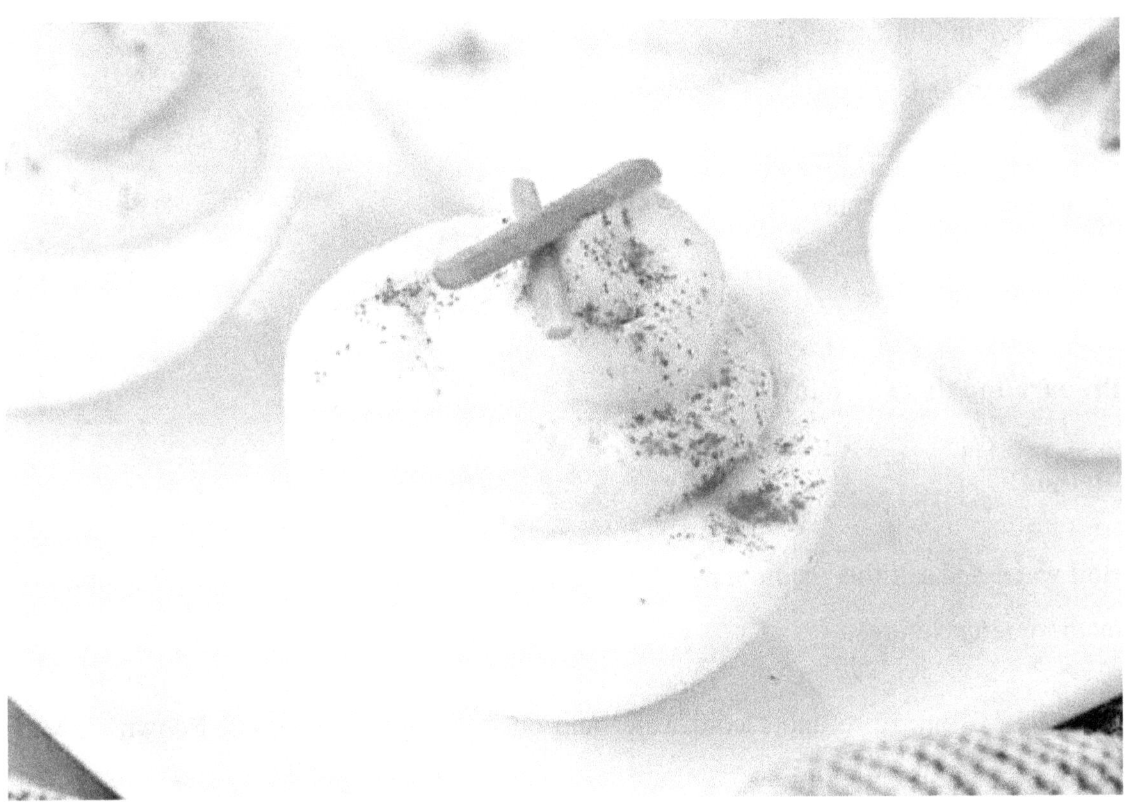

No matter what type of cooked eggs you decide to eat, as long as they are cooked, you are good to go! Eggs will offer pregnant women an excellent source of proteins and many vitamins and minerals, including choline, known to help your baby's brain development greatly.

Ingredients:

- 6 large eggs
- 1 minced green onion
- ½ cup sour cream
- 1 tsp. smoked paprika
- 2 Tbsp. sweet pickled relish
- Salt, black pepper

Servings: 6-12

Preparation time: 55 min

Method:

Boil water and salt in a medium pot. Carefully place the eggs and cook for 30 minutes on medium temperature.

Once time is up, rinse under cold water and once the eggs have cooled down enough, remove the shells carefully.

Slice each egg lengthwise and remove all egg yolks.

Place the yolks in a mixing bowl and place the white parts on a serving plate.

In the mixing bowl, add the rest of the ingredients and mash up together.

Fill each egg halves with the mixture and add some minced parsley if you like to decorate.

Refrigerate any leftovers.

15. Seriously tasty lentils patties

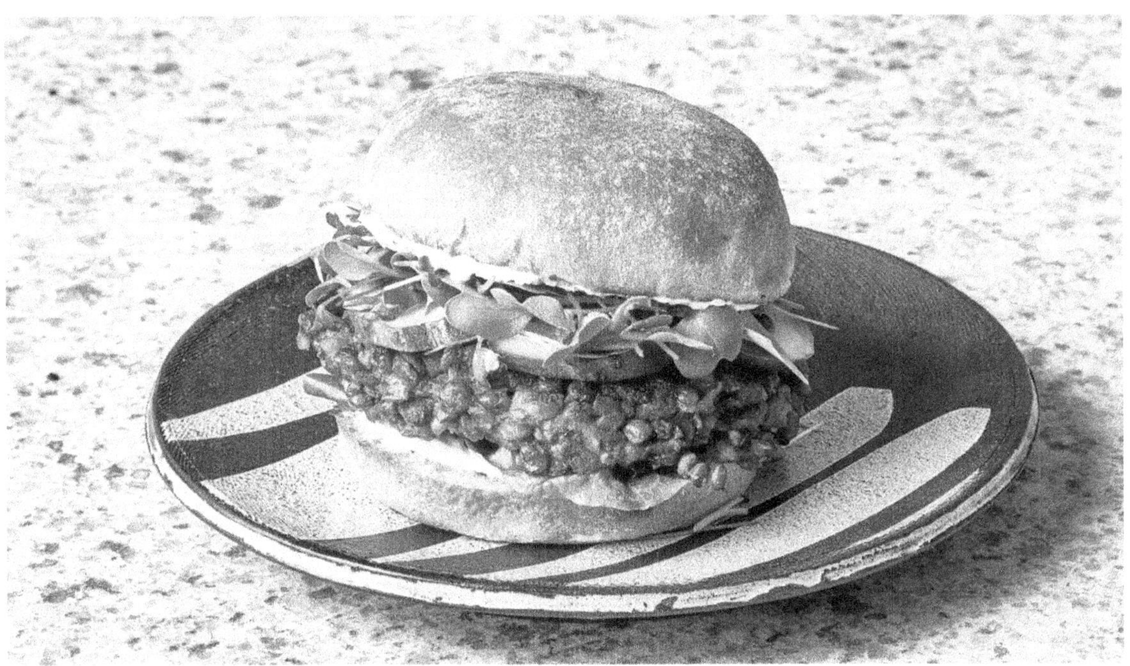

As we said before, you can add beans to your regular diet while you are pregnant. Lentils are full of proteins, folate, and vitamins. You will appreciate how tasty these lentils patties are, you will adopt them even after your pregnancy is over! You can serve these patties on buns and make sandwiches. In that case, I would use the thin bagels or perhaps pita bread. I have also crumbled the patties before and serve them on top of a salad.

Ingredients:

- 2 cans cooked lentils
- 1 cup seasoned breadcrumbs
- 1 shredded peeled medium carrot
- ½ tsp. ground turmeric
- ½ tsp. ground cumin
- Salt, black pepper
- 1 Tbsp. lemon juice
- 1 large egg
- 1 tbsp. sour cream
- Oliver oil for cooking

Servings: 4

Preparation time: 25 min

Method:

Rinse and drain carefully the lentils and lemon juice and place them in the container of your blender.

Activate until it is reduced in a paste.

Then dump the mixture into a mixing bowl.

Add the rest of the ingredients and combine them with your hands.

Form 4 patties.

Heat in a large skillet the olive oil on medium temperature and fry the patties for about 20 minutes.

Serve with your favorite dipping sauce, preferably one made with a yoghurt base.

16. Fruits and nuts on a bed of greens

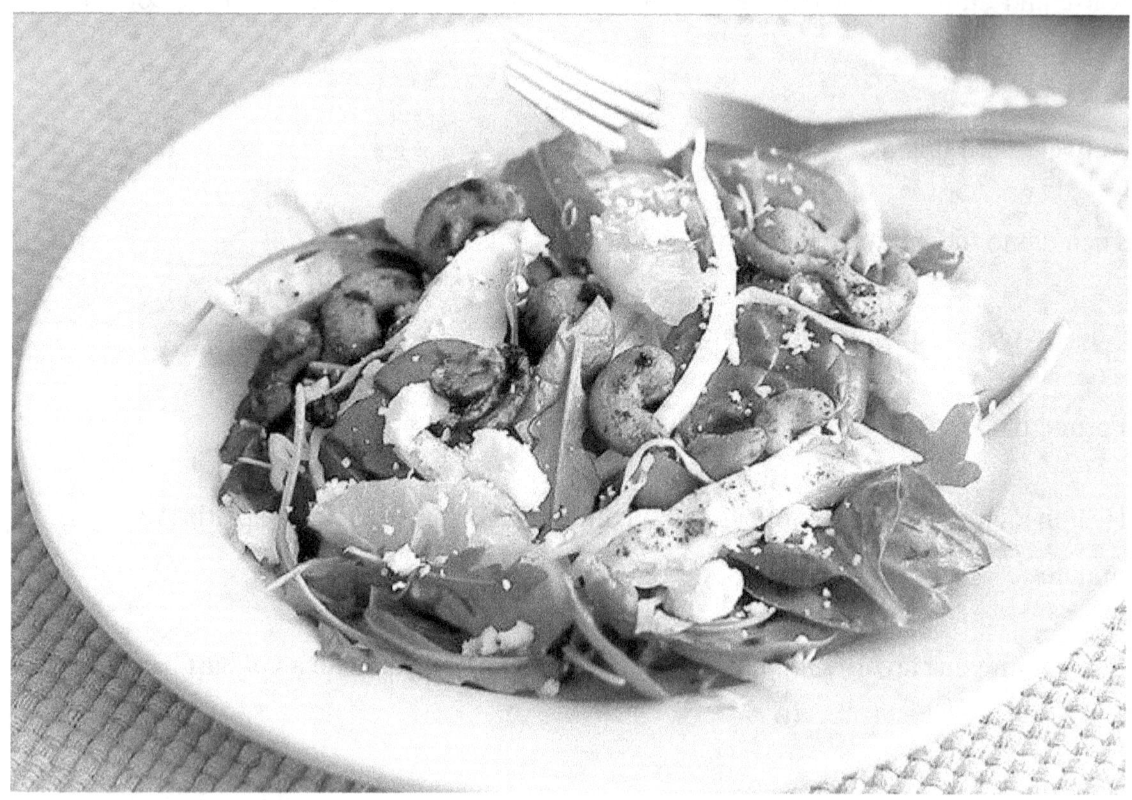

In this salad, we are combining nuts, fruits, and cheese, 3 foods we suggest to add in your diet during your pregnancy. You can also vary the type of fruits, nuts, and cheese you prefer to use, stay away from the soft cheese we listed previously.

Ingredients:

- 4-6 cups favorite greens, I usually choose a mixture of spinach and arugula leaves for this recipe
- 3-4 fresh organs, peeled and sectioned
- 2 tbsp. diced red onion
- ½ cup chopped cashews
- 1 cup shredded Mozzarella cheese
- Vinaigrette with no raw eggs, please verify the labels correctly (I often just pick a raspberry balsamic vinegar)
- Cooked chicken or turkey leftovers (optional)

Servings: 4

Preparation time: 15 min

Method:

In a large mixing bowl, combine the greens, red onion, nuts and cheese.

Add the vinaigrette and toss everything together.

Divide the mixture into 4 plates or bowls.

Add the orange slices and meat if you choose to.

Enjoy!

17. Asparagus and peppers on pasta

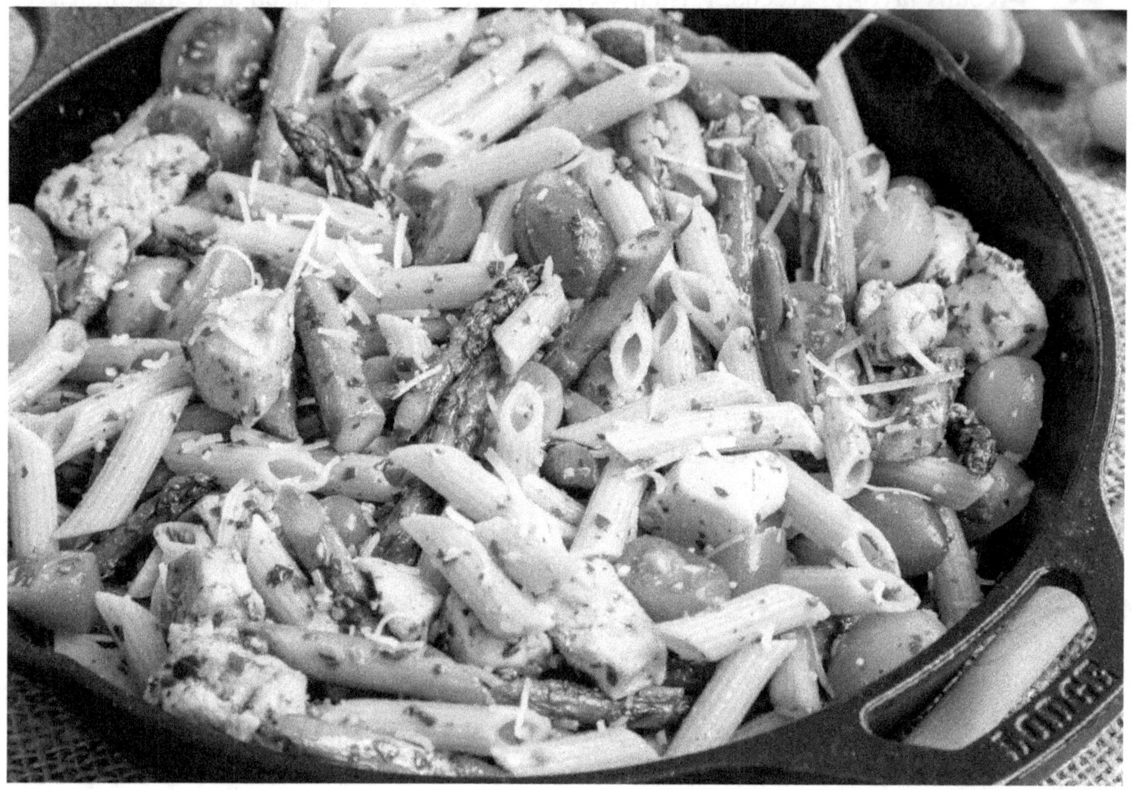

Pregnant or not, I do love asparagus! They are dark green, so you can only imagine how recommendable they are for you. They are actually packed with iron, vitamin K, and folate. They are super tasty, and you should try to grill them sometimes also, they turn out terrific. Don't forget to use your very favorite type of pasta; it makes even more enjoyable.

Ingredients:

- 1 pound fresh asparagus
- 1 large sliced red bell pepper
- 1 small yellow onion
- 1 Tbsp. minced garlic
- 1 cup pesto sauce
- 1 tbsp. lemon juice
- 1 box pasta of your choice: fettuccini or rotini or other
- 1 ½ cups shredded Parmesan cheese
- Fresh minced parsley when serving

Servings: 4

Preparation time: 40 min

Method:

Boil water and salt in a large saucepan for the noodles.

In a second pot, boil water as well to steam cook the asparagus.

While the paste and asparagus are cooking, both for about 12 minutes, let us sauté the veggies.

In a large skillet, heat the oil and cook the onion, garlic and peppers.

When the pasta is done, drain well and dump in the skillet with the cooked veggies.

Also, add the pesto sauce and lemon juice and mix together.

Lastly, drain the asparagus well, cut the hard ends and cut them in about 3 pieces each.

Add also to the pasta dish and mix.

Taste and adjust with salt and pepper if you think it is needed.

Serve for lunch or dinner with Parmesan cheese on top.

18. Awesome homemade hummus

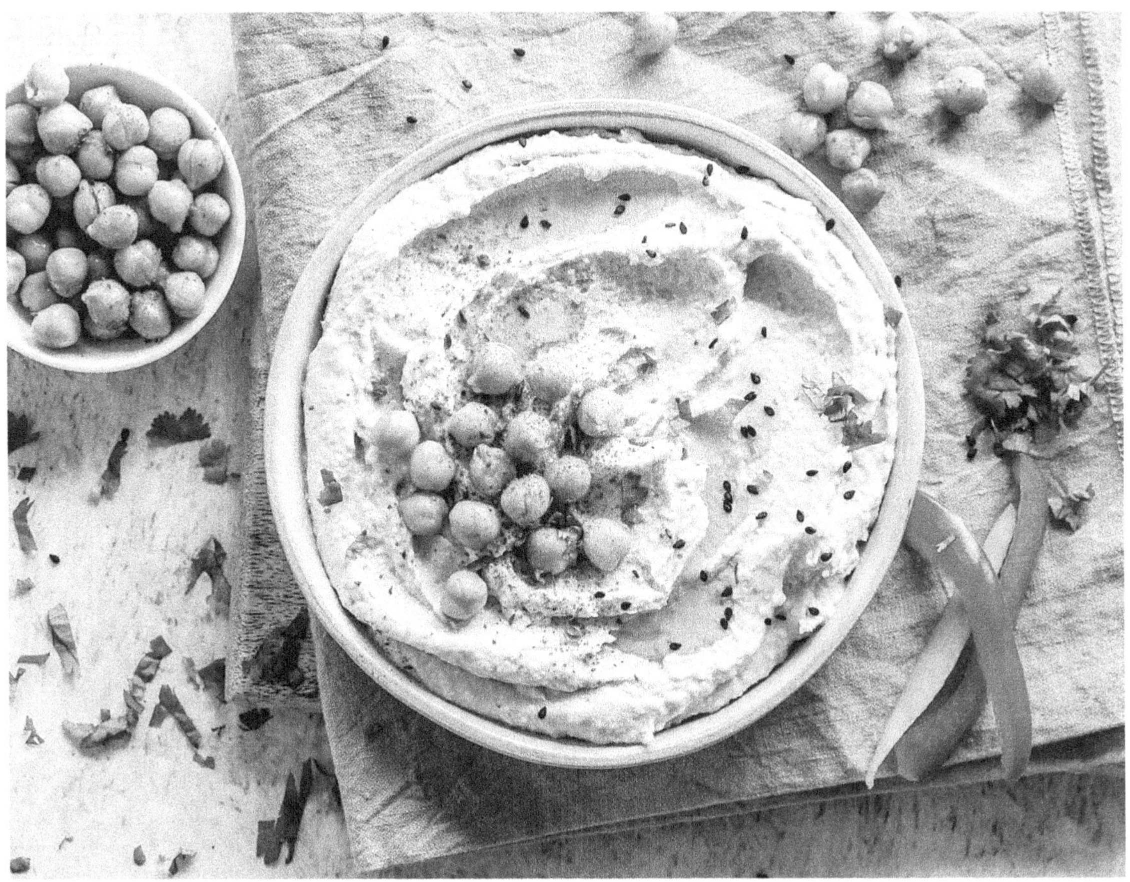

You can purchase hummus from the store, the one that already made. However, nothing like homemade hummus as you can control the exact used **Ingredients**, including healthy chickpeas for you and your baby. If you can't find the tahini butter or oil, please don't worry, you can use some olive or avocado oil.

Ingredients:

- 2 cans chickpeas
- 2 tbsp. tahini butter
- 1 Tbsp. olive oil
- 2 tbsp. raw cashews
- 1 Tbsp. minced garlic
- Salt, pepper
- 1 Tbsp. minced fresh parsley
- 1 Tbsp. lime juice
- Pita chips, celery sticks, carrots stick when serving

Servings: 4-6

Preparation time: 15 min

Method:

Use a coffee or nuts grinder and reduce the cashews into dust. Set aside.

In the blender's container, combine together the lemon juice, oil, tahini butter, grinded cashews, garlic, seasonings.

Activate until the texture is completely smooth.

Dump into a lovely serving container and add some fresh parsley to decorate.

Refrigerate any leftovers.

19. Vegetarian stew for pregnant ladies

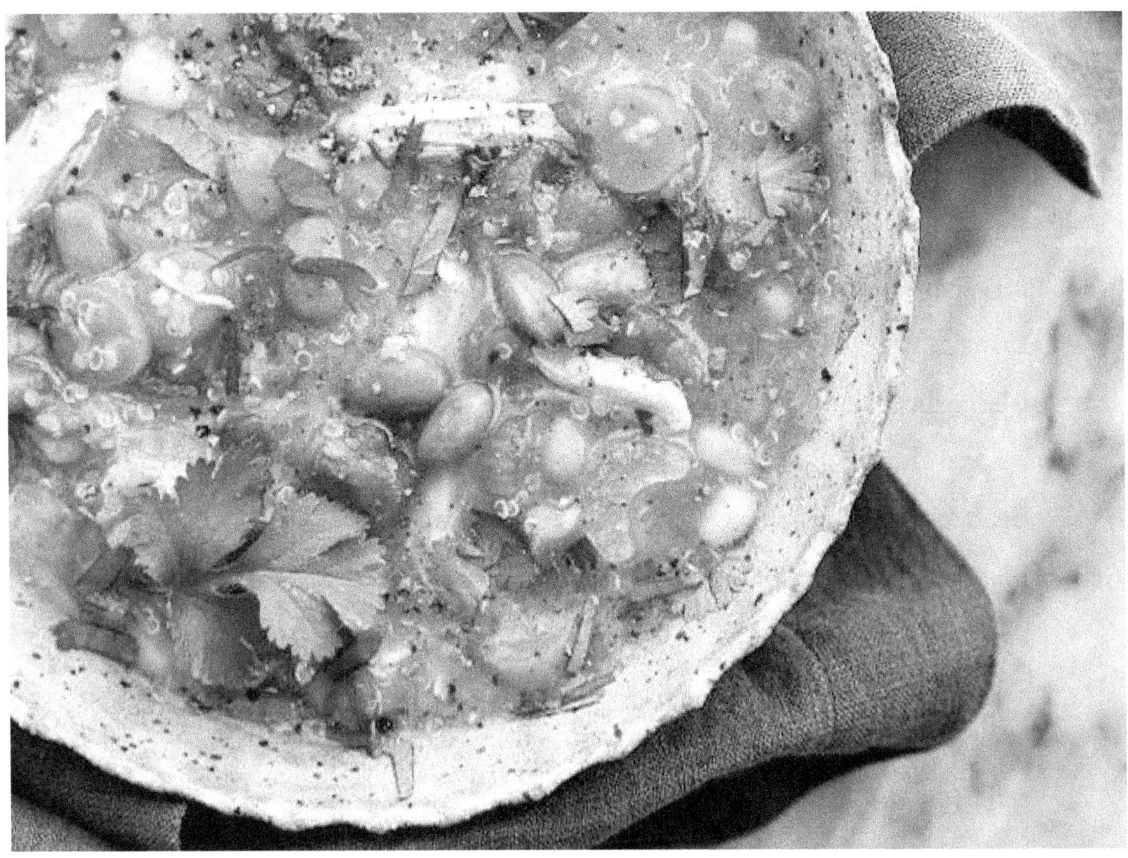

More beans please! This colorful recipe will please you. You can use the beans you prefer; I prefer to add black and red. As you already know by now, beans are an excellent choice during pregnancy; you will get a large amount of proteins from them. This recipe stayed with me after my pregnancy was over because I love it, and it is also so easy to make.

Ingredients:

- 2 cans black beans
- 2 cans red kidney beans
- 1 can sweet corn
- 5 cups turkey broth
- ¼ cup fresh minced herbs including: parsley, basil, oregano and thyme
- 1 Tbsp. minced garlic
- 1 small diced red onion
- 1 large diced carrots
- 1 sliced zucchini
- 1 can tomato sauce
- 1 large can crushed tomatoes
- 1 Tbsp. tomato paste
- Salt, pepper
- 1 tsp. chili powder
- Olive oil

Servings: 4-6

Preparation time: 60 min

Method:

You can make this recipe use your stovetop and a large saucepan or you can also decide to use the crockpot.

Either one the next few steps will be the same.

Heat oil in a skillet and sautéed together the garlic, onion, carrot, zucchini and season with salt and pepper.

Meanwhile, open, rinse and drain all the beans and set aside.

Let us use the slow cooker this time.

Add the cooked veggies, beans, broth, seasonings, corn, tomatoes, tomato sauce, and tomato paste in the slow cooker.

Set the temperature to low and keep cooking for 4 hours.

Mid-way, you should check on the stew and taste and adjust the seasonings if you want to.

Serve with sour cream, cheese on top or any additional topping you prefer.

20. Extremely healthy vegetables soup

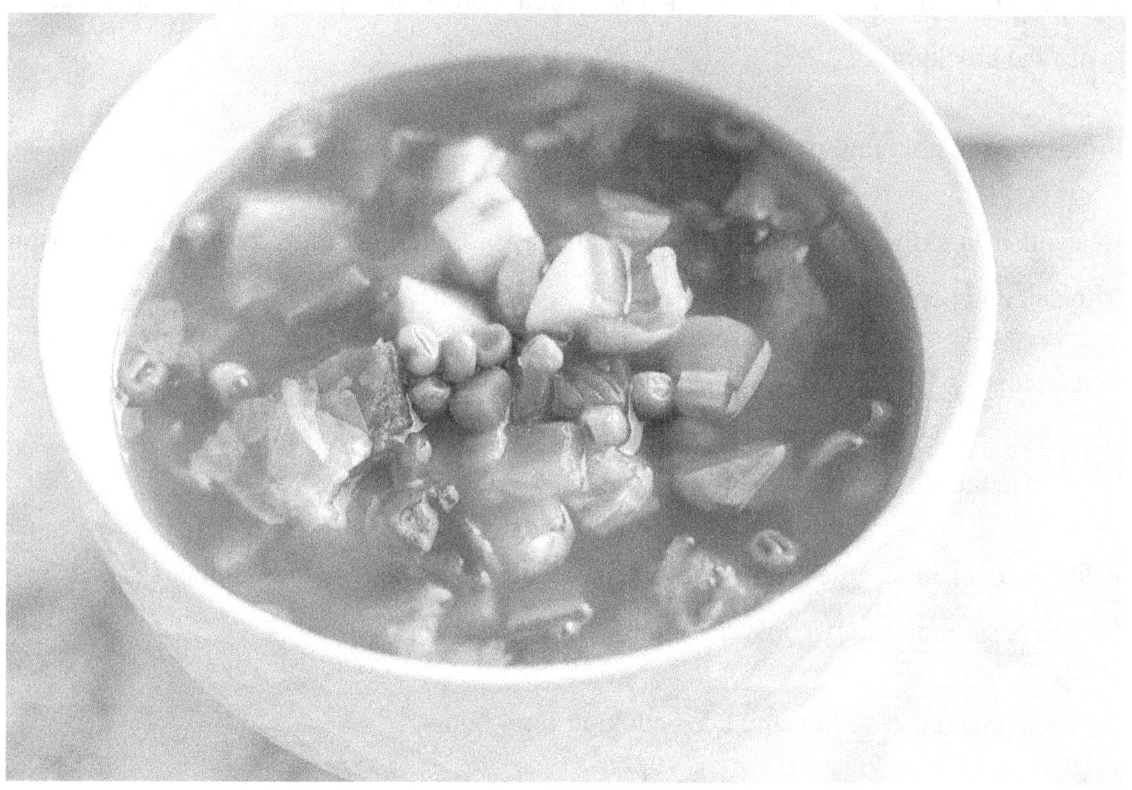

Again, this recipe should be one of your go-to recipes, no matter if you are pregnant or not! Get ready for a lot of flavors and goodness in one bowl! Vegetables are an undeniable source of vitamins, minerals, fiber, and antioxidants. You can use your veggies that might go bad soon and cook them in your soup! We will also add rice to the soup, and it makes it even more of a complete meal for hungry moms.

Ingredients:

- 2 cups green chopped cabbage
- 1 chopped turnip
- 1 large sliced carrot
- 3 cups chopped kale
- 1 small chopped sweet onion
- 2 large chopped sweet potatoes
- 1 large canned
- 1 tsp. ground cumin
- 1 tbsp. Italian seasonings
- Salt, black pepper
- 1 can gumbo soup
- 1 ½ cups white rice
- 6 cups vegetables broth

Servings: 4-6

Preparation time: 60 min

Method:

You should use a large saucepan for this recipe.

Also, in a medium pot, boil water and pre-cook the turnip, carrot and sweet potatoes for 10 minutes.

Heat some butter or oil in the largest pot and sautéed the garlic, onion and cabbage for 10 minutes.

Once the boiled veggies are done, drain well land add to the other ones and cook another 5 minutes, adding salt and pepper.

Then dump the broth and the gumbo soup.

You might wonder why a can of gumbo soup. Honest, it reminds me of my childhood, and I think the seasoning they include is special.

Add the remaining seasonings and the rice and bring to boil.

Once the soup is boiling, place on medium-low temperature and continue cooking for 30 minutes at least.

The rice will be done, you can then lower the temperature to low and let the soup simmer for a while.

Serve in your favorite soup bowls and with your favorite crackers or bread.

21. Green but delicious smoothie

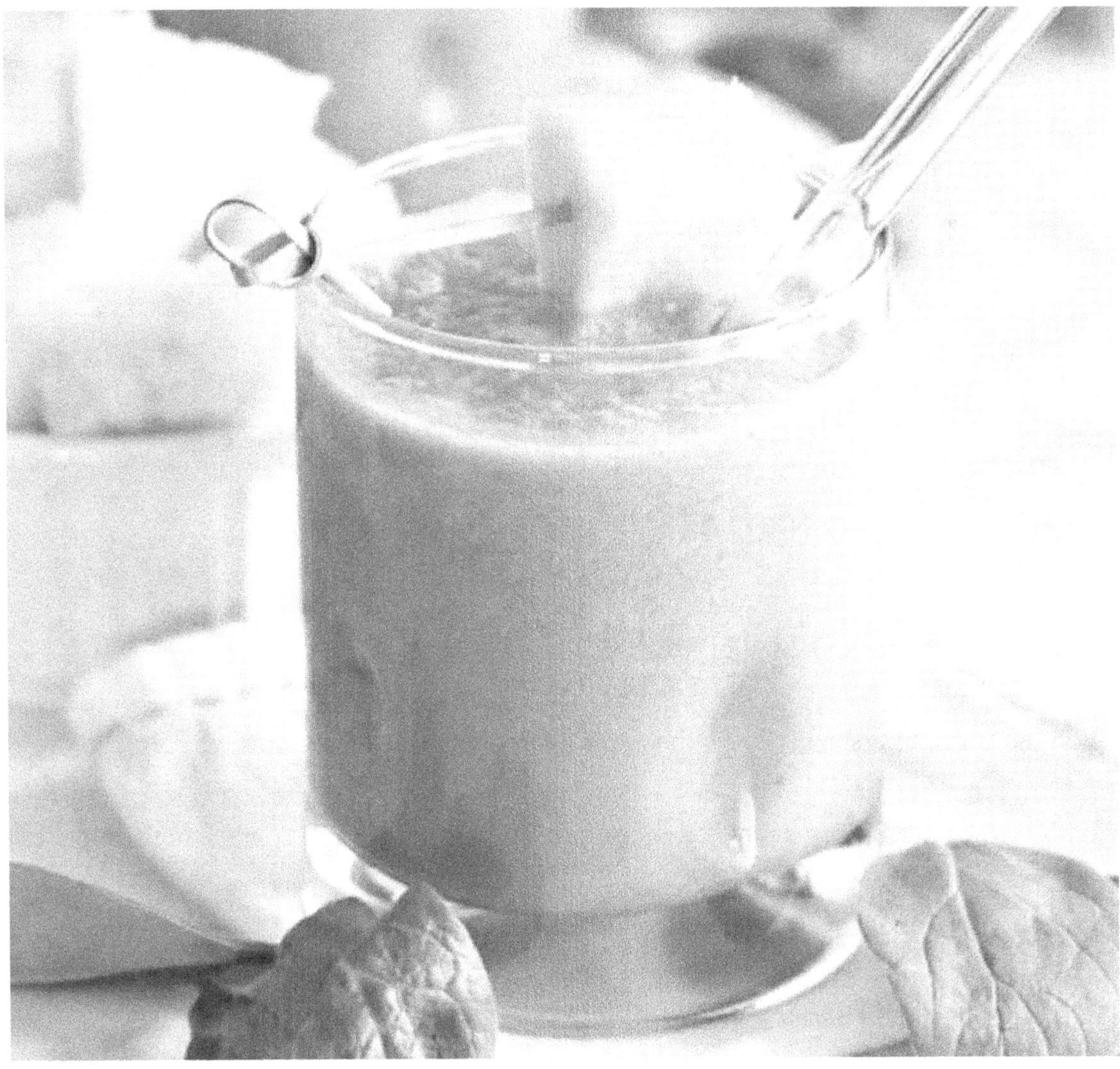

Green drinks can be a little scary. We are simply not quite used to sip on the green stuff. However, please do not let the color intimidate you and taste it! I guarantee that this concoction is full of deliciousness and vitamins! Please feel free to replace the spinach by kale, or any other dark leafy vegetable of your choice.

Ingredients:

- 1 cup fresh baby spinach leaves
- 1 cup plain Greek yoghurt
- 1 cup diced pineapple
- 1 green apple, chopped
- 1 Tbsp. vanilla proteins powder of your choice
- 1 cup coconut milk

Servings: 2

Preparation time: 10 min

Method:

Get your blender out and 2 tall glasses.

Chop the fruits, I personally leave the apple's skin, it is full of vitamins.

Combine the milk, proteins powder, pineapple, apple, yoghurt and spinach in the blender.

Activate a few times for 1 minute or so, or until the texture is perfect for a smoothie.

Pour into 2 separate glasses.

If I am alone I still make double the recipe so I can keep it for alter and add a little lemon juice to keep the smoothie form turned brown.

22. Spaghetti sauce served on zucchini noodles

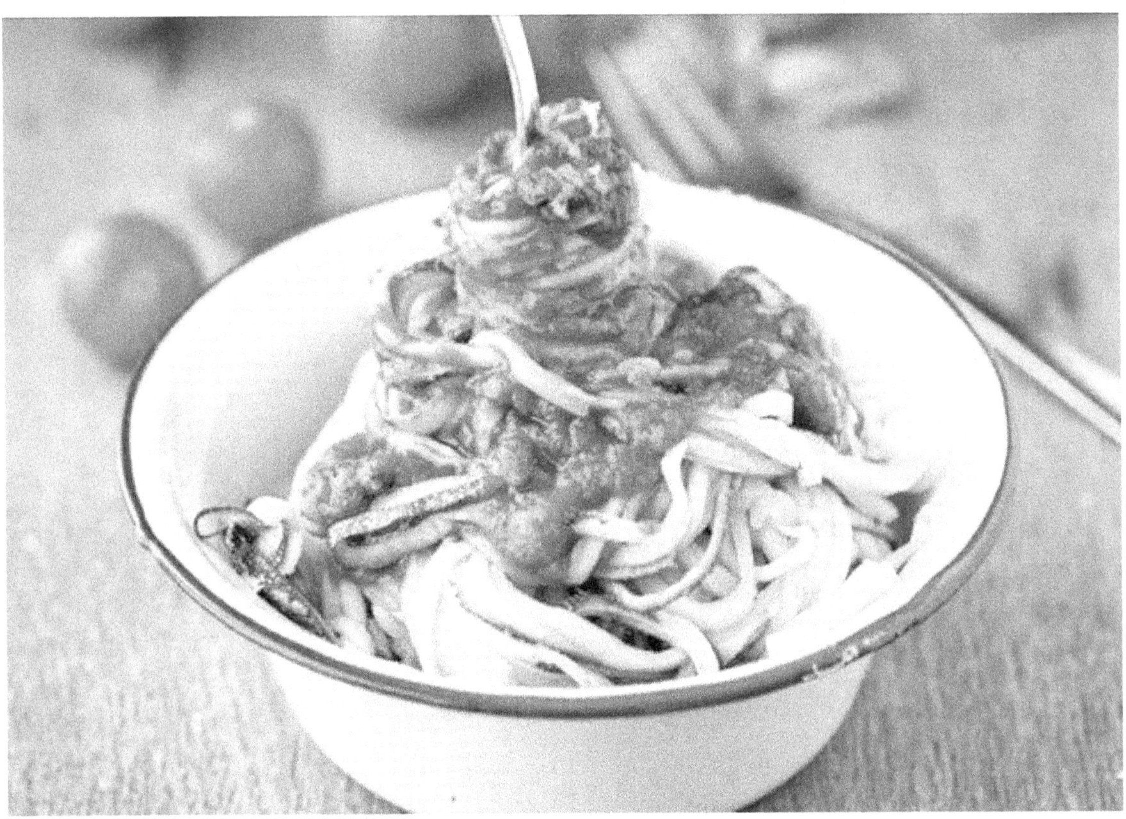

No matter what sauce you prefer to use for your spaghetti, usually, you can certainly use with zucchinis noodles. You will keep your dish overall low in carbs and high in fiber and vitamins. I love using pesto sauce sometimes. Zucchinis give you an excellent amount of manganese, vitamin C, vitamin A, fiber, folate, copper, and phosphorous. Enjoy!

Ingredients:

- 2-3 medium zucchinis
- Sea salt
- Olive oil

Sauce

- 1 1/2 pounds Grass fed ground beef
- 1 Tbsp. minced garlic
- 2 cups button mushrooms, sliced
- 1 small chopped green bell pepper
- 1 small chopped sweet onion
- 1 large can crushed tomatoes
- 1 small can tomato paste
- 1 medium can tomato sauce
- 1 Tbsp. Italian seasonings
- Salt, black pepper

Servings: 4

Preparation time: 1 hour

Method:

Let us prepare the sauce first. I insist you on choosing a high quality ground beef. Although we mentioned that red meat is good for you, you do not want to take any chances on getting poor quality ground beef or high fat meat. So, choose wisely.

In a skillet, heat a little oil and cook the ground meat, adding some salt and pepper. It should take up to 20 minutes, make sure it is done and remove excess fat.

In a large saucepan, heat some oil and cook the onion, garlic, pepper and mushrooms for 10 minutes.

Remove any excess oil. Add the cooked meat, tomatoes, tomato sauce, tomato paste and all seasonings.

Let that sauce simmer while you cook the zucchini noodles. Unlike regular pasts, you do not need to boil water. Use a skillet and heat some olive oil and add the noodles. Add a little oil. Cook for about 4 minutes on medium high.

Get your plates or bowls ready and divide the noodles and sauce in 4 portions.

Enjoy with or without Parmesan cheese on top.

23. Broccoli and mushrooms yummy casserole

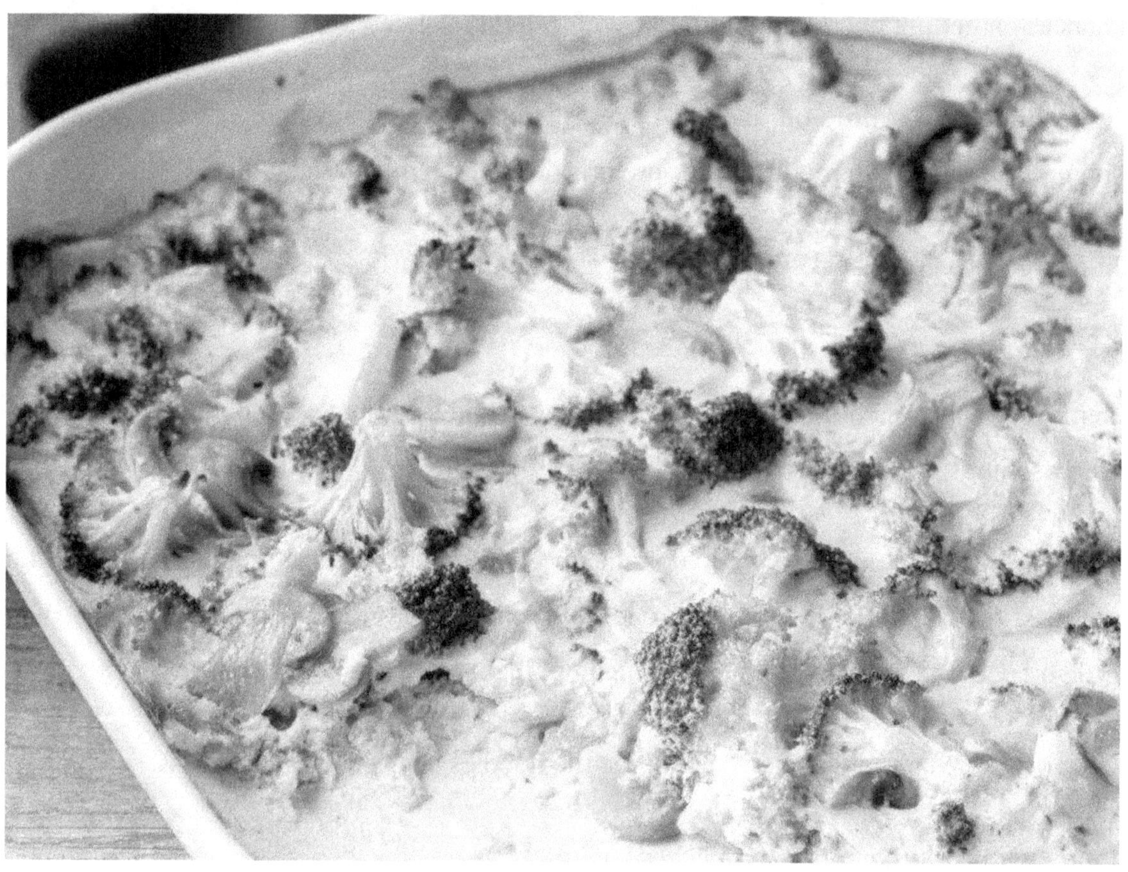

In a casserole, you can add so many healthy ingredients, so go for it, create your next casserole. Let us inspire you. We love to add broccoli because, as a dark green vegetable, it gives you fiber, vitamins C, K, A, calcium, and iron. In addition, it is rich in antioxidants.

Ingredients:

- 3 cups broccoli florets (fresh or thawed if you choose frozen ones)
- 2 cups fresh cauliflower florets
- 2 cups fresh button mushrooms
- 1 Tbsp. minced garlic
- 1 small chopped yellow onion
- 1 can mushrooms soup
- 11/2 cups shredded sharp cheddar cheese
- 1 cup ½ whole milk
- ½ cup sour cream
- ½ tsp. ground cumin
- ½ tsp. dried oregano
- Salt, black pepper
- Pinch smoked paprika on top
- Butter

Servings: 4-6

Preparation time: 50 min

Method:

Preheat the oven to 375 degrees F.

Grease a medium rectangle baking dish and set aside.

Steam cook the broccoli and cauliflower florets for just a little over 5 minutes to give them a jumpstart. Drain well and place in a large mixing bowl.

Sautéed the onion, garlic and mushrooms in butter in a large skillet for 10 minutes also.

Add to the mixing bowl, along with the cream of mushrooms, milk, sour cream and seasonings.

Combine well before dumping into the greased dish.

Add a layer of Cheddar cheese and sprinkle some smoked paprika on top.

Place in the oven to cook for 40 minutes.

Serve as a side dish with any grilled meat.

24. Stuffed potato with cottage cheese mix

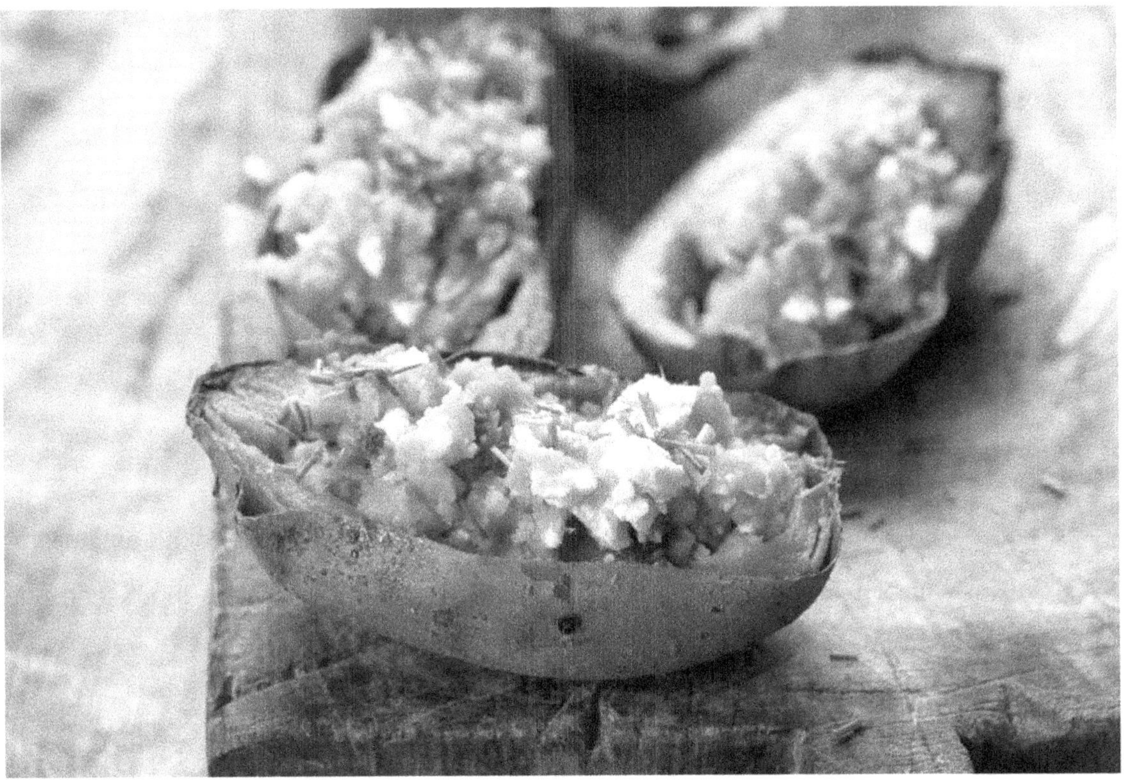

This might be the perfect afternoon snack or evening snack for any pregnant ladies. The sweet potato is more nutritious than regular white potatoes and certainly tastier. It contains beta-carotene and vitamin A. In addition, it is a great source of fiber. Adding cottage cheese in it will help you add that additional texture and avoid high-fat cheeses you may normally use.

Ingredients:

- 1 large sweet potato
- 2 Tbsp. cottage cheese
- Pinch cinnamon
- 1 tsp. butter

Servings: 1

Preparation time: 10 min

Method:

Let's make one potato at a time. It would be totally fine for you to bake the potatoes in the oven instead of using the microwave. Especially if you are making more than one potato, it makes total sense.

Get all ingredients out. Wash the potato and place it on a microwave dish in the microwave to cook for 4-6 minutes on high temperature, depending on size of potato.

When done, cut open lengthwise, and remove the flesh.

Place the flesh of the potato in a mixing bowl and add the butter and cinnamon and mix well.

Place the mixture back into the potato and ad the cottage cheese on top.

Microwave again if you think it got too cold to eat.

25. Brussels sprouts warm salad

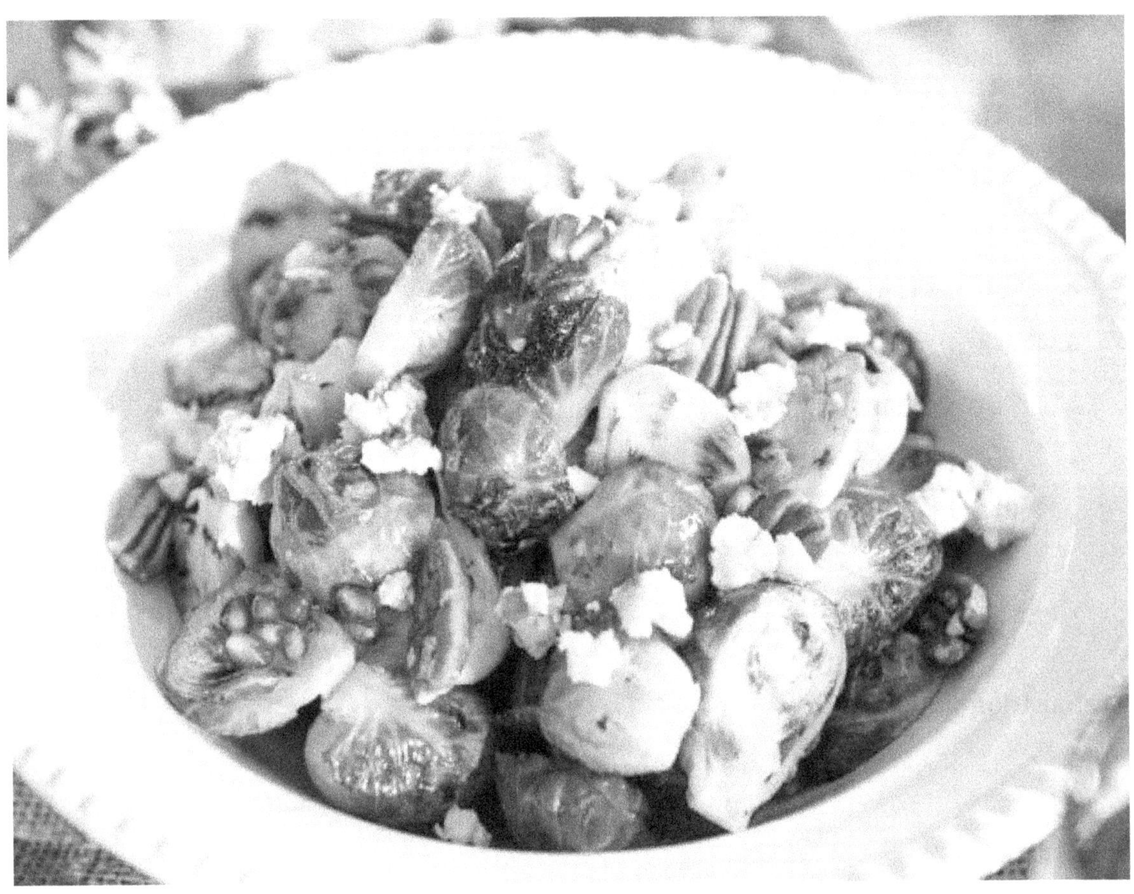

Here is our Grande finale, a Brussel sprouts warm dish. During your pregnancy, it is safe to eat Brussel sprouts. You should eat them in moderation and make sure they cook thoroughly. Follow our lead!

Ingredients:

- 2 pounds fresh Brussels sprouts (you could also use some frozen ones, thawed for recipe)
- 2 Tbsp. unsalted butter
- 1 cup chopped pecans
- 2 tbsp. maple syrup
- 2 Tbsp. diced red onions
- 1 Tbsp. minced garlic
- ½ tsp. cayenne pepper
- Pinch cinnamon
- Sea salt

Servings: 4

Preparation time: 45 min

Method:

Start by cooking the Brussels sprouts. I prefer to simply use boiling water with salt and cook them until done. We will sauté them again so if they are still slightly firm, that's okay.

In a large skillet or a wok, heat butter and cook the garlic, onion and Brussel sprouts together.

Sprinkle the cinnamon and cayenne pepper and add the apply syrup.

Stir often and add finally the chopped nuts. Make sure all ingredients are well combined and serve warm.

It is really surprising how a sweet touch to Brussels sprouts makes all the different, even your children might enjoy this recipe!

Conclusion

Let's talk some additional nutritional advices you could benefit from during your pregnancy:

You should take some prenatal vitamins. Follow your doctor's orders, but in most cases, you will benefit from them. They normally should provide the following: folic acid, vitamin D, vitamin C, calcium, thiamine, and riboflavin. It is also possible that you might benefit from iron or magnesium.

You do not need to eat for 2 during your pregnancy. This is a myth. Will your appetite increase? Most likely, yes! However, you should not double-up all your portions. It is important to eat a healthy balanced diet during your pregnancy to avoid gaining too much weight but also avoid developing gestational diabetes or other complications. Your baby is counting on you. You should ingest, in average, only about 300 calories more a day during your pregnancy months.

In order to keep your diet balanced, make sure you ingest the right type of calories. We already gave you an overview of healthy and safe food to consume during pregnancy, so make sure you follow that guideline. You should gain between 25 and 35 pounds normally total during your 9 months of pregnancy. More specifically, you need to get enough proteins, as it will directly affect the growth of your baby. You should also get up to 50% more iron intake than usual when you are pregnant. Do not spare the calcium either, your baby needs it as you need it, so your bones stay strong throughout the pregnancy.

During your pregnancy, you should drink enough water for sure but avoid, of course, the alcohol and caffeine as we talked about. You can drink milk and 100% fruit juices also.

We hope we contribute to making your pregnancy a little easier or even better a little healthier. Make sure you continue reading about nutrition while you are breastfeeding as well. Congratulations and Bon appetite!

About the Author

Ivy's mission is to share her recipes with the world. Even though she is not a professional cook she has always had that flair toward cooking. Her hands create magic. She can make even the simplest recipe tastes superb. Everyone who has tried her food has astounding their compliments was what made her think about writing recipes.

She wanted everyone to have a taste of her creations aside from close family and friends. So, deciding to write recipes was her winning decision. She isn't interested in popularity, but how many people have her recipes reached and touched people. Each recipe in her cookbooks is special and has a special meaning in her life. This means that each recipe is created with attention and love. Every ingredient carefully picked, every combination tried and tested.

Her mission started on her birthday about 9 years ago, when her guests couldn't stop prizing the food on the table. The next thing she did was organizing an event where chefs from restaurants were tasting her recipes. This event gave her the courage to start spreading her recipes.

She has written many cookbooks and she is still working on more. There is no end in the art of cooking; all you need is inspiration, love, and dedication.

Author's Afterthoughts

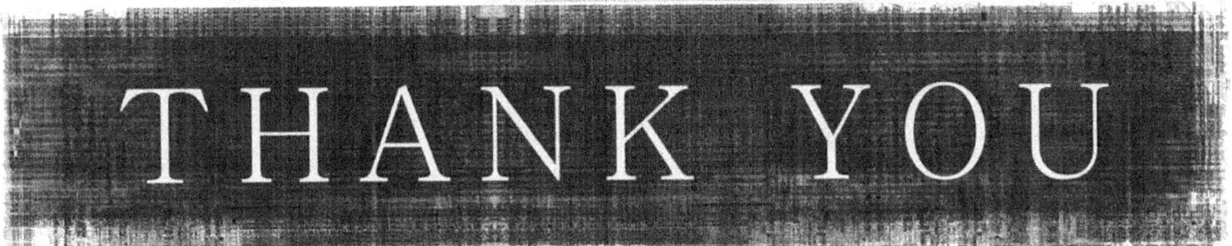

I am thankful for downloading this book and taking the time to read it. I know that you have learned a lot and you had a great time reading it. Writing books is the best way to share the skills I have with your and the best tips too.

I know that there are many books and choosing my book is amazing. I am thankful that you stopped and took time to decide. You made a great decision and I am sure that you enjoyed it.

I will be even happier if you provide honest feedback about my book. Feedbacks helped by growing and they still do. They help me to choose better content and new ideas. So, maybe your feedback can trigger an idea for my next book.

Thank you again

Sincerely

Ivy Hope